BRIGHT F[UTURES]

Guidelines for Health[y]
Infants, Children, an[d]

MW01004437

THIRD EDITION

POCKET GUIDE

Editors

Joseph F. Hagan, Jr, MD, FAAP
Judith S. Shaw, RN, MPH, EdD
Paula M. Duncan, MD, FAAP

FUNDED BY
US Department of Health and Human Services
Health Resources and Services Administration
Maternal and Child Health Bureau

PUBLISHED BY
The American Academy of Pediatrics

CITE AS

Hagan JF, Shaw JS, Duncan P, eds. 2008. *Bright Futures: Guidelines for Health Supervision of Infants, Children, and Adolescents,* Third Edition. *Pocket Guide.* Elk Grove Village, IL: American Academy of Pediatrics.

Library of Congress Catalog Card Number: 2007929964
ISBN-13: 978-1-58110-224-6
ISBN-10: 1-58110-224-0

BF0027

PUBLISHED BY
American Academy of Pediatrics
141 Northwest Point Blvd
Elk Grove Village, IL 60007-1098
USA
847-434-4000
AAP Web site: www.aap.org
Bright Futures Web site: http://brightfutures.aap.org

Additional copies of this publication are available from the American Academy of Pediatrics Online Bookstore at www.aap.org/bookstore.

This publication has been produced by the American Academy of Pediatrics under its cooperative agreement (U06MC00002) with the US Department of Health and Human Services, Health Resources and Services Administration (HRSA), Maternal and Child Health Bureau (MCHB).

TABLE OF CONTENTS

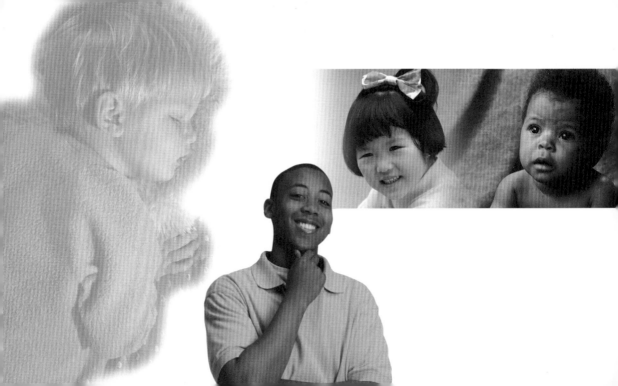

Bright Futures at the American Academy of Pediatrics

Founded in 1930, the American Academy of Pediatrics (AAP) is an organization of 60,000 pediatricians who are committed to the attainment of optimal physical, mental, and social health and well-being for all infants, children, adolescents, and young adults.

The Bright Futures initiative was launched in 1990 under the leadership of the Federal Maternal and Child Health Bureau (MCHB) of the Health Resources and Services Administration (HRSA) to improve the quality of health services for children through health promotion and disease prevention. In 2002, the MCHB selected the AAP to lead the Bright Futures initiative. With the encouragement and strong support of the MCHB, the AAP and its many collaborating partners set out to update the *Bright Futures Guidelines* as a uniform set of recommendations for health care professionals. The *Bright Futures Guidelines* are the cornerstone of the Bright Futures initiative and the foundation for the development of all Bright Futures materials.

What Is Bright Futures?
Bright Futures is a set of principles, strategies, and tools that are theory based, evidence driven, and systems oriented that can be used to improve the health and well-being of all children through culturally appropriate interventions that address their current and emerging health promotion needs at the family, clinical practice, community, health system, and policy levels.

Goals of Bright Futures
- Enhance health care professionals' knowledge, skills, and practice of developmentally appropriate health care in the context of family and community.
- Promote desired social, developmental, and health outcomes of infants, children, and adolescents.
- Foster partnerships between families, health care professionals, and communities.
- Increase family knowledge, skills, and participation in health-promoting and prevention activities.
- Address the needs of children and youth with special health care needs through enhanced identification and services.

For more information about Bright Futures and available materials and resources, visit http://brightfutures.aap.org.

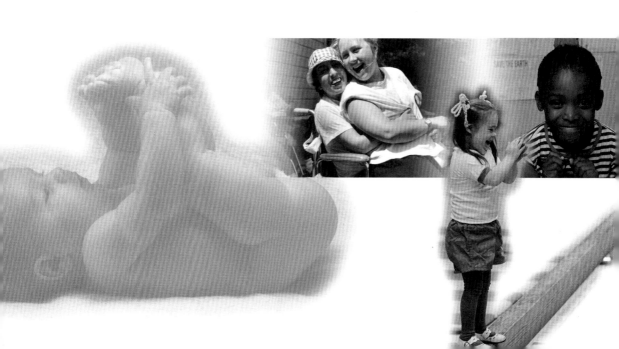

How to Use This Guide

The *Pocket Guide* is based on *Bright Futures: Guidelines for Health Supervision of Infants, Children, and Adolescents,* Third Edition. Presenting key information from the Guidelines, the *Pocket Guide* serves as a quick reference tool and training resource for health care professionals.

Sections of the Pocket Guide

Themes: Highlights 10 cross-cutting child health topics that are discussed in depth in the Guidelines. These themes are important to families and health care professionals in their mission to promote the health and well-being of all children. The *Pocket Guide* lists these themes; see the Guidelines for the full text.

The Health Visit: Focuses on specific age-appropriate health and developmental issues.

Visit Priorities: The Bright Futures Expert Panels acknowledge that the most important priority is to attend to the concerns of the parent or youth. In addition, they have developed 5 priority health supervision topics for each visit.

Developmental Observation: Includes observation of parent-child interaction, developmental surveillance, and school performance questions.

Physical Exam: Recommends a complete physical exam, including specific issues for each visit.

Screening: Includes universal and selective screening procedures and risk assessment.

Immunizations: Provides Centers for Disease Control and Prevention/National Immunization Program and American Academy of Pediatrics *Red Book* Web sites for current schedules.

Anticipatory Guidance: Presents guidance for families, organized by the 5 priorities of each visit. Sample questions also are provided for selected topics. Guidance and questions in **black** type are intended for the parent; guidance and questions in **green** type are intended for the child/adolescent/young adult. These can be modified to match the health care professional's communication style.

Appendices: Includes developmental milestones at-a-glance charts for infancy and early childhood, a chart on social and emotional development in middle childhood, a chart on domains of adolescent development, recommended medical screening tables, a tooth eruption chart, a sexual maturity ratings chart, and a list of useful Web sites.

Core Concepts

In today's complex and changing health care system, health care professionals can improve the way they carry out each visit by using an innovative health promotion curriculum developed specifically to help professionals integrate Bright Futures principles into clinical practice.

This unique curriculum, developed by a health promotion work group supported by the Maternal and Child Health Bureau, includes 6 core concepts:

- Partnership
- Communication
- Health promotion/illness prevention
- Time management
- Education
- Advocacy

A summary of each of these core concepts is presented on the following pages to help all professionals, both those in training and experienced practitioners, bring Bright Futures alive and make it happen for children and families. For more information about this unique health promotion curriculum, visit www.pediatricsinpractice.org.

All 6 core concepts rely on the health care professionals' skills in using open-ended questions to communicate effectively, partner with and educate children and their families, and serve as their advocates to promote health and prevent illness in a time-efficient manner.

Open-ended questions

- Help to start a conversation
- Ask: "Why?" "How?" "What?"
- Are interpretive
- Have a wide range of possible answers
- Stimulate thinking
- Promote problem solving

EXAMPLES:

- *How do you and your partner manage the baby's behavior? What do you do when you disagree?*
- (To a child) *Tell me about your favorite activities at school.*

Techniques

- Begin with affirming questions.

EXAMPLE:

- *"What are some games you're really good at?"*
- Wait at least 3 seconds to allow the family to respond to the question.
- Ask questions in a supportive way to encourage communication.

Building Effective Partnerships

A clinical partnership is a relationship in which participants join together to ensure health care delivery in a way that recognizes the critical roles and contributions of each partner (child, family, health care professional, and community) in promoting health and preventing illness. Following are 6 steps for building effective health partnerships:

1. Model and encourage open, supporting communication with child and family.
- Integrate family-centered communication strategies.
- Use communication skills to build trust, respect, and empathy.

2. Identify health issues through active listening and "fact finding."
- Selectively choose Bright Futures Anticipatory Guidance questions.
- Ask open-ended questions to encourage more complete sharing of information.
- Communicate understanding of the issues and provide feedback.

3. Affirm strengths of child and family.
- Recognize what each person brings to the partnership.
- Acknowledge and respect each person's contributions.
- Commend family for specific health and developmental achievements.

4. Identify shared goals.
- Promote view of health supervision as partnership between child, family, health care professional, and community.
- Summarize mutual goals.
- Provide links between stated goals, health issues, and available resources in community.

5. Develop joint plan of action based on stated goals.
- Be sure that each partner has a role in developing the plan.
- Keep plan simple and achievable.
- Set measurable goals and specific timeline.
- Use family-friendly negotiation skills to ensure agreement.
- Build in mechanism and time for follow-up.

6. Follow up to sustain the partnership.
- Share progress, successes, and challenges.
- Evaluate and adjust plan.
- Provide ongoing support and resources.

Fostering Family-Centered Communication

Effective Behaviors
- Greet each family member and introduce self.
- Use names of family members.
- Incorporate social talk in the beginning of the interview.
- Show interest and attention.
- Demonstrate empathy.
- Appear patient and unhurried.
- Acknowledge concerns, fears, and feelings of child and family.
- Use ordinary language, not medical jargon.
- Use Bright Futures Anticipatory Guidance questions.
- Give information clearly.
- Query level of understanding and allow sufficient time for response.
- Encourage additional questions.
- Discuss family life, community, and school.

Active Listening Skills: Verbal Behaviors
- Allow child and parents to state concerns without interruption.
- Encourage questions and answer them completely.
- Clarify statements with follow-up questions.
- Ask about feelings.
- Acknowledge stress or difficulties.
- Allow sufficient time for a response (wait time >3 seconds).
- Offer supportive comments.
- Restate in the parent's or child's words.
- Offer information or explanations.

Active Listening Skills: Nonverbal Behaviors
- Nod in agreement.
- Sit down at the level of the child and make eye contact.
- Interact with or play with the child.
- Show expression, attention, concern, or interest.
- Convey understanding and empathy.
- Touch child or parent (if appropriate).
- Draw pictures to clarify.
- Demonstrate techniques.

Promoting Health and Preventing Illness

Because families often hesitate to begin discussion, it is essential that health care professionals identify and focus on the individual needs of the child and family.

1. Identify relevant health promotion topics.

- Ask open-ended, nonjudgmental questions to obtain information and identify appropriate guidance.
- Ask specific follow-up questions to communicate understanding and focus the discussion.

EXAMPLE:

- *"How often and for how long do you breastfeed the baby? How do you know when he wants to be fed?"*

- Listen for verbal, and observe nonverbal, cues to discover underlying or unidentified concerns.

EXAMPLE:

- *"How do you balance your roles of partner and parent? When do you make time for yourself?"*

Note:

- If parent hesitates with an answer, try to determine the reason.
- If parent brings in child multiple times for minor problems, explore the possibility of another unresolved concern.

2. Give personalized guidance.

- Introduce new information and reinforce healthy practices.

EXAMPLES:

- *Take time for self and partner for leisure and exercise.*
- *Encourage partner to help care for child.*
- *Accept support from friends, family.*

3. Incorporate family and community resources.

- Approach child within context of family and community.
- Identify each family member's role.

EXAMPLES:

- *"Tell me about your child's bedtime routine."*
- *"Who's responsible for household chores?"*

- Identify community resources, such as a lactation consultant or local recreation centers.
- Develop working relationships with community professionals and establish lines of referral.
- Create a list of local resources with contact information.

4. Come to closure.

- Be sure that the health message is understood.

EXAMPLES:

- *"Have I addressed your question?"*
- *"Do you have any other concerns about your teen's health?"*

- Identify possible barriers.

EXAMPLE:

- *"What problems do you think you might have in following through with what we discussed today?"*

Managing Time for Health Promotion

1. Maximize time for health promotion.

- Use accurate methods that minimize documentation time.
- Ask family to complete forms in waiting area.
- Organize chart in consistent manner.
- Scan chart before meeting with child and family.
- Train staff to elicit information and provide follow-up with family.

2. Clarify health care professional's goals for visit.

- Review screening forms and other basic health data.
- Observe parent-child interaction.
- Identify needs, then rank them in order of importance.
- Clarify visit priorities.

Note:

The *Pocket Guide* organizes each visit's Anticipatory Guidance by designated priorities.

3. Identify family's needs and concerns for visit.

- Selectively use Bright Futures Anticipatory Guidance sample questions.
- Include open-ended questions to draw family into visit.

EXAMPLE:

- *"Tell me about the baby's sleeping habits. What position does she sleep in?* (Elicits more than yes/no answer and presents "teachable moment" on "back to sleep" and sudden infant death syndrome.)

4. Work with the family to prioritize goals for the visit.

- Explain purpose of visit (identify and address specific concerns and overall health and development).
- Identify family's and health care professional's shared goals.
- Prioritize needs through family-friendly negotiation.

EXAMPLE:

- *"I appreciate your concerns about _____. While you are here, I would also like to talk about _____."*

5. Suggest other options for addressing unmet goals.

- Acknowledge importance of issues that could not be fully addressed during the visit.
- Offer additional resources (handouts, CDs, videotapes/DVDs, Web-based materials).
- Suggest a follow-up visit or phone call.
- Provide referral to professional or community resource.

Educating Families Through Teachable Moments

Teachable moments occur multiple times each day, but often go unrecognized. Health supervision visits present opportunities for the health care professional to teach the child and family.

1. Recognize teachable moments in health visit.
2. Clarify learning needs of child and family.
3. Set a limited agenda and prioritize needs together.
4. Select teaching strategy.
5. Seek and provide feedback.
6. Evaluate effectiveness of teaching.

Four characteristics of the teachable moment

- Provides "information bites" (small amounts of information)
- Is directed to the child's or family's specific needs
- Is brief (eg, a few seconds)
- Requires no preparation time

TEACHING STRATEGIES	ADVANTAGES
•Telling (explain, provide information, give direction)	Works well when giving initial explanations or clarifying concepts
•Showing (demonstrate, model, draw)	Illustrates concepts for visual learners
•Providing resources (handouts, videos/DVDs, Web sites)	Serves as a reference after family leaves the office/clinic
•Questioning (ask open-ended questions, allow time for response)	Promotes problem solving, critical thinking; elicits better information; stimulates recall
•Practicing (apply new information)	Reinforces new concepts
•Giving constructive feedback (seek family's perspective, restate, clarify)	Affirms family's knowledge; corrects misunderstandings

Advocating for Children, Families, and Communities

Health care professionals can be involved in advocacy either at an individual level (eg, obtaining services for a child or family) or at a local or national level (eg, speaking with the media, community groups, or legislators).

1. Identify family needs or concerns.

- Use open-ended questions to identify specific needs or concerns of the family.

EXAMPLE:
   - *"What are some of the main concerns in your life right now?"*

- Choose a specific area of focus.

EXAMPLE:
   - *Obtaining special education services for a child.*

- Clarify family's beliefs and expectations about the issue.
- Determine what has been done to date, and what has (or hasn't) worked.

EXAMPLE:
   - *Parents may have tried unsuccessfully to obtain services for their child.*

- Obtain data through some initial "fact finding."

EXAMPLE:
   - *Contact board of education or local public health department.*

- Talk with others; determine progress.

EXAMPLE:
   - *Do any local school coalitions address this issue?*

2. Assess the situation.

- Determine existing community resources.
- Learn about existing laws that address the issue.
- Review the data and resources to be sure they support the issue.
- Assess political climate to determine support or opposition.

EXAMPLE:
   - *Is this issue of interest to anyone else (eg, school/early intervention teacher, local policy makers)? Who (or what) might oppose the advocacy efforts? Why?*

3. Develop a strategy.

- Limit efforts to a specific issue.

EXAMPLE:
   - *Obtaining special education services for one child rather than changing the laws for all.*

- Use existing resources.
- Start with small steps, then build upon successes.

4. Follow through.

- Be passionate about the issue, but willing to negotiate.
- Review the outcome.
- Evaluate your efforts.
- Determine next steps with family.
- Recognize that health care professionals and families can learn from one another about effective advocacy.

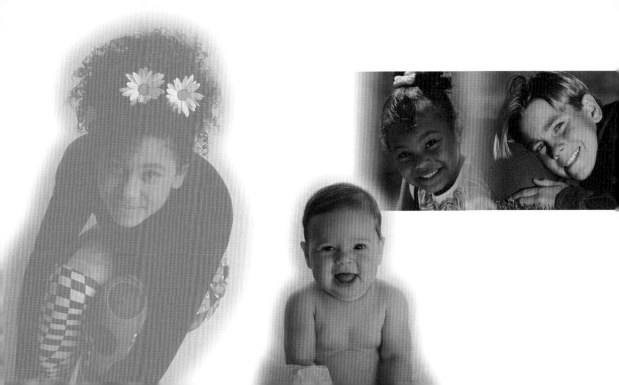

Supporting Families Successfully

Understanding and building on the strengths of families requires health care professionals to combine well-honed clinical interview skills with a willingness to learn from families. Families demonstrate a wide range of beliefs and priorities in how they structure daily routines and rituals for their children and how they use health care resources. This edition of the *Bright Futures Guidelines* places special emphasis on 3 areas of vital importance to caring for children and families.

Children and Youth With Special Health Care Needs
As of 2000, more than 9 million children in the United States have special health care needs. This means that 1 of every 5 households includes a child with a developmental delay, chronic health condition, or some form of disability. Family-centered care that promotes strong partnerships and honest communication is especially important when caring for children and youth with special health care needs. These children and youth now live normal life spans and tend to require visits with health care professionals more frequently than other children.

At the same time, the impact of *specialness* or extensive health care needs should not overshadow the *child*.

The child or youth with special health care needs shares most health supervision requirements with her peers. Bright Futures uses screening, ongoing assessment, health supervision, and anticipatory guidance as essential interventions to promote wellness and identify differences in development, physical health, and mental health for all children.

Cultural Competence
Cultures form around language, gender, disability, sexual orientation, religion, or socioeconomic status. Even people who have been fully acculturated within mainstream society can maintain values, traditions, communication patterns, and child-rearing practices of their original culture. Immigrant families, in particular, face many cultural stressors.

It is important for health care professionals who serve children and families from backgrounds other than their own to listen and observe carefully, learn from the family, and work to build trust and respect. If possible, the presence of a staff member who is familiar with a family's community and fluent in the family's language is helpful during discussions with families.

Complementary and Alternative Care

Families must be empowered as care participants. Their unique ability to choose what is best for their children must be recognized. The health care professional must be aware of the disciplines or philosophies that are chosen by the child's family, especially if the family chooses a therapy that is unfamiliar or outside the scope of standard care. Such therapies are not necessarily harmful or without potential benefit. Providers of standard care need not be threatened by such choices. Therapies can be safe and effective, safe and ineffective, or unsafe.

The use of complementary and alternative care is particularly common when a child has a chronic illness or condition. Parents are often reluctant to tell their health care professional about such treatments, fearing disapproval. Health care professionals should ask parents directly, in a nonjudgmental manner, about the use of complementary and alternative care.

Consultation with colleagues who are knowledgeable about complementary and alternative care might be necessary. Discussion with a complementary and alternative care therapist also may be useful.

Bright Futures Themes

A number of themes are of key importance to families and health care professionals in their common mission to promote the health and well-being of children from birth through adolescence. These themes are:

- Promoting Family Support
- Promoting Child Development
- Promoting Mental Health
- Promoting Healthy Weight
- Promoting Healthy Nutrition
- Promoting Physical Activity
- Promoting Oral Health
- Promoting Healthy Sexual Development and Sexuality
- Promoting Safety and Injury Prevention
- Promoting Community Relationships and Resources

The *Bright Futures Guidelines* provide an in-depth, state-of-the-art discussion of these themes, with evidence regarding effectiveness of health promotion interventions at specific developmental stages from birth to early adulthood. Health care professionals can use these comprehensive discussions to help families understand the context of their child's health and support their child's and family's development.

Because of the overwhelming importance to overall health and well-being of mental health and healthy weight, and the prevalence of problems in these areas, the Bright Futures authors have designated Promoting Mental Health and Promoting Healthy Weight as **Significant Challenges to Child and Adolescent Health** for this edition.

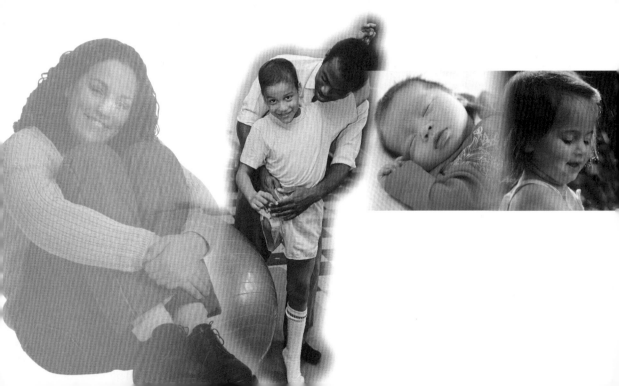

Bright Futures Health Supervision Visits

This section presents all the Bright Futures Visits from the Prenatal Visit to the 21 Year Visit. The Table below lists the acronyms used in this section.

ACRONYMS USED IN THE BRIGHT FUTURES HEALTH SUPERVISION VISITS	
AAP	American Academy of Pediatrics
ATV	All-terrain vehicle
BMI	Body mass index
CBE	Clinical breast examination
CDC	Centers for Disease Control and Prevention
CPR	Cardiopulmonary resuscitation
DVD	Digital Versatile Disc
HIV	Human immunodeficiency virus
IEP	Individualized Education Program
OTC	Over-the-counter
SMR	Sexual maturity rating
STI	Sexually transmitted infection
TV	Television
WIC	The Special Supplemental Nutrition Program for Women, Infants, and Children

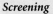

Observation of Parent-Child Interaction: Who asks questions and who provides responses to questions? (Observe parent with partner, other children, other family members.) Do the verbal and nonverbal behaviors/communication among family members indicate support and understanding, or differences of opinion and conflicts?

Screening

Discuss the purpose and importance of the newborn screening tests (metabolic, hearing) that will be done in the hospital before the baby is discharged.

Immunizations

Discuss routine initiation of immunizations.

Anticipatory Guidance

FAMILY RESOURCES

Family support systems, transition home (assistance after discharge), family resources, use of community resources

- Your family's health values/beliefs/practices are important to the health of your baby.
  What health practices do you follow to keep your family healthy?
- Anticipate challenges of caring for new baby.
- Ensure support systems at home (friends, relatives).
- Contact community resources for help, if needed.
  Tell me about your living situation. How are your resources for caring for the baby?

PARENTAL (MATERNAL) WELL-BEING

Physical/mental/oral health; nutritional status; medication use; pregnancy risks

- Maintain your health (medical appointments, vitamins, diet, sleep, exercise, personal safety).
  What have you been doing to keep yourself and your baby healthy? Do you always feel safe with your partner? Would you like information on where to go or who to contact if you ever need help?
- Know your HIV status.
- Consider your feelings about the pregnancy.
  How do you, your family, the father feel about your pregnancy? What works for communicating with each other/making decisions?

INFANCY | PRENATAL VISIT

Key= Guidance for parents, *questions*

BREASTFEEDING DECISION

Breastfeeding plans, breastfeeding concerns (past experiences, prescription or nonprescription medications/drugs, family support of breastfeeding), breastfeeding support systems, financial resources for infant feeding

- Choose breastfeeding if possible; use iron-fortified formula if formula feeding.
  What are your plans for feeding your baby?
- Tell me about supplement/OTC use.
- Contact WIC/community resources if needed.
  Are you concerned about having enough money to buy food or infant formula? Would you be interested in resources that would help you afford to care for you and your baby?

SAFETY

Car safety seats, pets, alcohol/substance use (fetal effects, driving), environmental health risks (smoking, lead, mold), guns, fire/burns (water heater setting, smoke detectors), carbon monoxide detectors/alarms

- Use safety belt.
- Install rear-facing car safety seat in back seat.
- Learn about pet risks.
  Do you have pets at home? If you have cats, have you been tested for toxoplasmosis antibodies?

- Don't use alcohol/drugs.
- Keep home/vehicle smoke-free; check home for lead, mold.
- Remove guns from home; if gun necessary, store unloaded and locked with ammunition separate.
  Do you keep guns at home? Are there guns in homes you visit (grandparents, relatives, friends)?
- Set home water temperature <120°F; install smoke detectors, carbon monoxide detector/alarm.

NEWBORN CARE

Introduction to the practice, illness prevention, sleep (back to sleep, crib safety, sleep location), newborn health risks (hand washing, outings)

- Ask for information about practice.
- Put baby to sleep on back; choose crib with slats $\leq 2\frac{3}{8}$" apart; have baby sleep in your room, in own crib.
- Wash hands frequently (diaper changes, feeding).
- Limit baby's exposure to others.

Observation of Parent-Child Interaction: Do parents recognize and respond to the baby's needs? Are they comfortable when feeding, holding, or caring for the baby? Do they have visitors or other signs of a support network?

Surveillance of Development: Has periods of wakefulness, is responsive to parental voice and touch, is able to be calmed when picked up, looks at parents when awake, moves in response to visual or auditory stimuli.

Physical Exam. Complete, including: Measure and plot length, weight, head circumference; plot weight-for-length. Assess/Observe alertness, distress, congenital anomalies; skin lesions or jaundice; head shape/size, fontanelles, signs of birth trauma; eyes/eyelids, ocular mobility. Examine pupils for opacification, red reflexes.

Assess/Observe pinnae, patency of auditory canals, pits or tags; nasal patency, septal deviation; cleft lip or palate, natal teeth, frenulum; heart rate/rhythm/sounds, heart murmurs. Palpate femoral pulses. Examine/Determine umbilical cord/cord vessels; descended testes, penile anomalies, anal patency. Note back/spine/foot deformities. Perform Ortolani and Barlow maneuvers. Detect primitive reflexes.

Screening (See p 58.)

Universal: Metabolic and Hemoglobinopathy; Hearing
Selective: Blood Pressure; Vision

Immunizations

CDC: www.cdc.gov/vaccines
AAP: www.aapredbook.org

Anticipatory Guidance

FAMILY READINESS

Family support, maternal wellness, transition, sibling relationships, family resources

- Accept help from family, friends.
- Never hit or shake baby.
  What makes you get upset with the baby? What do you do when you get upset?

- Take care of yourself; make time for yourself, partner.
- Feeling tired, blue, or overwhelmed in first weeks is normal. If it continues, resources are available for help.
- Community agencies can help.
  Tell me about your living situation. What are your resources for caring for the baby?

INFANT BEHAVIORS

Infant capabilities, parent-child relationship, sleep (location, position, crib safety), sleep/wake states (calming)

4

Key= Guidance for parents, *questions*

- Learn baby's temperament, reactions.
- Create nurturing routines; physical contact (holding, carrying, rocking) helps baby feel secure.
- Put baby to sleep on back; don't use loose, soft bedding; have baby sleep in your room, in own crib.

FEEDING

Feeding initiation, hunger/satiation cues, hydration/jaundice, feeding strategies (holding, burping), feeding guidance (breastfeeding, formula)

- Exclusive breastfeeding during the first 4-6 months provides ideal nutrition, supports best growth and development; iron-fortified formula is recommended substitute; recognize signs of hunger, fullness; develop feeding routine; adequate weight gain = 6-8 wet diapers a day, no extra fluids; cultural/family beliefs.
- *If breastfeeding:* 8-12 feedings in 24 hours; continue prenatal vitamin; avoid alcohol.
- *If formula feeding:* Prepare/store formula safely; feed every 2-3 hours; hold baby semi-upright; don't prop bottle.
- Contact WIC/community resources if needed.
  Are you concerned about having enough money to buy food for yourself or infant formula?

SAFETY

Car safety seats, tobacco smoke, falls, home safety (review of priority items if no prenatal visit was conducted)

- Rear-facing car safety seat in back seat; never put baby in front seat of vehicle with passenger air bag. Baby must remain in car safety seat at all times during travel.
- Always use safety belt; do not drive under the influence of alcohol or drugs.
- Keep home/vehicle smoke-free.
- Keep hand on baby when changing diaper/clothes.
- Keep home safe for baby.
  What changes have you made in your home to ensure your baby's safety?

ROUTINE BABY CARE

Infant supplies, skin care, illness prevention, introduction to practice/early intervention referrals

- Use fragrance-free soap/lotion, avoid powders; avoid direct sunlight.
- Change diaper frequently to prevent diaper rash.
- Cord care: "air drying" by keeping diaper below; call if bad smell, redness, fluid from the area.
- Wash your hands often.
  What suggestions have you heard about things you can do to keep your baby healthy?
- Avoid others with colds/flu.

Observation of Parent-Child Interaction: Do parents and newborn respond to each other? Do parents appear content, depressed, angry, fatigued, overwhelmed? Are parents responsive to newborn's distress? Do the parents appear confident in caring for newborn? What are the parents' and newborn's interactions around comforting, dressing/changing diapers, and feeding? Do parents support each other?

Surveillance of Development: Is able to sustain periods of wakefulness for feeding, will gradually become able to establish longer stretch of sleep (4-5 hours at night); turns and calms to parent's voice, communicates needs through behaviors, has undifferentiated cry; is able to fix briefly on faces or objects, follows face to midline; is able to suck/swallow/breathe, shows strong primitive reflexes, lifts head briefly in the prone position.

Physical Exam. Complete, including: Measure and plot length, weight, head circumference. Plot weight-for-length. Assess/Observe rashes, jaundice, dysmorphic features; eyes/eyelids, ocular mobility. Examine pupils for opacification, red reflexes. Assess dacryocystitis. Ascult for heart murmurs. Palpate femoral pulses. Inspect umbilical cord/cord vessels. Perform Ortolani/Barlow maneuvers. Assess/Observe posture, neurologic tone, activity level, symmetry of movement, state regulation.

Screening (See p 58.)

Universal: Metabolic and Hemoglobinopathy; Hearing
Selective: Blood Pressure; Vision

Immunizations

CDC: www.cdc.gov/vaccines
AAP: www.aapredbook.org

Anticipatory Guidance

PARENTAL (MATERNAL) WELL-BEING

Health and depression, family stress, uninvited advice, parent roles

• Recognize fatigue, "baby blues." Rest and sleep when baby sleeps.

How is the adjustment to the new baby going? Are there times when you feel sad, hopeless, or overwhelmed?

• Accept help from partner, family, friends.
• Maintain family routines; spend time with your other children.
• Handle unwanted advice by acknowledging, then changing subject.

Key= Guidance for parents, *questions*

NEWBORN TRANSITION

Daily routines, sleep (location, position, crib safety), state modulation (calming), parent-child relationship, early developmental referrals

- Help baby to develop sleep and feeding routines. Put baby to sleep on back; choose crib with slats $\leq 2\frac{3}{8}$" apart, keep sides up; don't use loose, soft bedding; have baby sleep in your room, in own crib.
- Help baby wake for feeding by patting/diaper change/undressing.
- Calm baby with stroking head or gentle rocking.

NUTRITIONAL ADEQUACY

Feeding success (weight gain), feeding strategies (holding, burping), hydration/jaundice, hunger/satiation cues, feeding guidance (breastfeeding, formula)

- Exclusive breastfeeding during the first 4-6 months provides ideal nutrition, supports best growth and development; iron-fortified formula is recommended substitute; recognize signs of hunger, fullness; develop feeding routine; adequate weight gain = 6-8 wet diapers a day, no extra fluids; cultural/family beliefs.
  How do you know if your baby is hungry? Had enough to eat?
- *If breastfeeding:* Avoid own allergens; wait 1 month before offering pacifier.
  How is breastfeeding going? What concerns do you have?

- *If formula feeding:* Prepare/store formula safely; feed 2 oz every 2-3 hours and more if still seems hungry; hold baby semi-upright; don't prop bottle.
- Contact WIC/lactation consultant if needed.

SAFETY

Car safety seats, tobacco smoke, hot liquids (water temperature)

- Use rear-facing car safety seat in back seat; never put baby in front seat of vehicle with passenger air bag.
- Always use safety belt; do not drive under the influence of alcohol or drugs.
- Don't smoke; keep home/vehicle smoke-free.
- Avoid drinking hot liquids while holding baby; set home water temperature <120°F.

NEWBORN CARE

When to call (temperature taking), emergency readiness (CPR), illness prevention (hand washing, outings), skin care (sun exposure)

- Take temperature rectally, not by ear.
  What thermometer do you use? Do you know how to use it?
- Create emergency preparedness plan (first-aid kit, list of telephone numbers).
- Wash hands often; avoid crowds.
- Avoid sun, use children's sunscreen; ask if rash is a concern.

7

Observation of Parent-Child Interaction: Do parents appear content, depressed, angry, fatigued, overwhelmed? Do parents appear uncertain or nervous? How do the parent and infant interact? How do parents respond to the infant's cues? Do they appear to be comfortable with each other and with the baby?

Surveillance of Development: Responsive to calming actions when upset; able to follow parents with eyes, recognizes the parents' voices; has started to smile; is able to lift his head when on tummy.

Physical Exam. Complete, including: Measure and plot length, weight, head circumference. Plot weight-for-length. Assess/Observe positional skull deformities; red reflexes, eye color/intensity/clarity, opacities, clouding of cornea. Ascult for heart murmurs. Palpate femoral pulses. Search for abdominal masses. Note umbilicus healing. Perform Ortolani/Barlow maneuvers. Assess neurologic tone, attentiveness to visual and auditory stimuli.

Screening (See p 58.)

Universal: Metabolic and Hemoglobinopathy; Hearing
Selective: Blood Pressure; Vision; Tuberculosis

Immunizations

CDC: www.cdc.gov/vaccines
AAP: www.aapredbook.org

Anticipatory Guidance

PARENTAL (MATERNAL) WELL-BEING

Health (maternal postpartum checkup, depression, substance abuse), return to work/school (breastfeeding plans, child care)

- Have postpartum checkup; recognize "baby blues."
  How are your spirits? What are your best and most difficult times of day with the baby? Do you find you're drinking, using herbs, or taking drugs to help you feel better?
- Make back-to-work/school plans; plan for breastfeeding, child care.

FAMILY ADJUSTMENT

Family resources, family support, parent roles, domestic violence, community resources

- Contact community resources if needed.
  Tell me about your living situation. How are your resources for caring for your baby (heat, appliances, housing, knowledge, insurance, money)? Who helps you with the baby?
- Take time for self, partner.

8

Key= Guidance for parents, *questions*

- Ask for help with domestic violence.
  Do you always feel safe in your home? Has your partner or ex-partner ever hit you? Are you scared that you or other caretakers may hurt the baby? Would you like information on where to go and who to contact for help?
- Learn infant first-aid/CPR/temperature taking; know emergency telephone numbers; wash hands often.

INFANT ADJUSTMENT

Sleep/wake schedule, sleep position (back to sleep, location, crib safety), state modulation (crying, consoling, shaken baby), developmental changes (bored baby, tummy time), early developmental referrals

- Develop consistent sleep/feeding routines.
- Put baby to sleep on back; choose crib with slats $\leq 2\frac{3}{8}$" apart; don't use loose, soft bedding; have baby sleep in your room, in own crib; choose mesh playpen with weave $<\frac{1}{4}$"; never leave baby in with drop side down.
- Hold, cuddle, talk to baby often; calm baby by talking, patting, stroking, rocking; never shake baby.
- Start "tummy time" when awake.

FEEDING ROUTINES

Feeding frequency (growth spurts), feeding choices (types of foods/fluids), hunger cues, feeding strategies (holding, burping), pacifier use (cleanliness), feeding guidance (breastfeeding, formula)

- Exclusive breastfeeding during the first 4-6 months is ideal; iron-fortified formula is recommended substitute; recognize signs of hunger, fullness; develop feeding routine; adequate weight gain = 5-8 wet diapers a day, 3-4 stools a day; burp at natural breaks; no extra fluids, food; recognize growth spurts.
  How do you know if your baby is hungry?
- *If breastfeeding:* Continue prenatal vitamin; wait until 4-6 weeks before offering pacifier/bottle.
- *If formula feeding:* Prepare/store formula safely; feed 2 oz every 2-3 hours and more if still seems hungry; hold baby semi-upright; don't prop bottle.

SAFETY

Car safety seats, toys with loops and strings, falls, tobacco smoke

- Use rear-facing car safety seat in back seat; never put baby in front seat of vehicle with passenger air bag.
- Always use safety belt; do not drive under the influence of alcohol or drugs.
- Keep hand on baby when changing diaper/clothes; keep bracelets, toys with loops, strings/cords away from baby.
- Don't smoke; keep home/vehicle smoke-free.

9

Observation of Parent-Child Interaction: How responsive are parents and infant to each other? Do parents appear content, depressed, angry, fatigued, overwhelmed? Are parents comfortable and confident with the infant? What are the parent-infant interactions around feeding/eating, comforting, and responding to infant cues? Do parent and partner support each other?

Surveillance of Development: Attempts to look at parent, smiles, is able to console and comfort self; begins to demonstrate differentiated types of crying, coos, has clearer behaviors to indicate needs. Indicates boredom; is able to hold up head and begins to push up in prone position, has consistent head control in supported sitting position, shows symmetrical movements of head, arms, and legs, shows diminishing newborn reflexes.

Physical Exam. Complete, including: Measure and plot length, weight, head circumference. Plot weight-for-length. Assess/Observe rashes or bruising, fontanelles; eyes/eyelids, ocular mobility, pupil opacification, red reflexes; heart murmurs, femoral pulses. Perform Ortolani/Barlow maneuvers. Assess torticollis, neurologic tone, strength and symmetry of movements.

Screening (See p 58.)

Universal: Metabolic and Hemoglobinopathy; Hearing
Selective: Blood Pressure; Vision

Immunizations

CDC: www.cdc.gov/vaccines
AAP: www.aapredbook.org

Anticipatory Guidance

PARENTAL (MATERNAL) WELL-BEING

Health (maternal postpartum checkup and resumption of activities, depression), parent roles and responsibilities, family support, sibling relationships

• Have postpartum checkup; talk with partner about family planning.

• Take time for self, partner; maintain social contacts.
• Engage other children in care of baby, as appropriate.

INFANT BEHAVIOR

Parent-child relationship, daily routines, sleep (location, position, crib safety), developmental changes, physical activity (tummy time, rolling over, diminishing newborn reflexes), communication and calming

10

Key= Guidance for parents, *questions*

- Hold, cuddle, talk/sing to baby.
  What do you and your partner enjoy most about your baby? What is challenging?
- Maintain regular sleep/feeding routines.
- Put baby to sleep on back; choose crib with slats $\leq 2\frac{3}{8}$" apart, keep sides up; don't use loose, soft bedding; have baby sleep in your room, in own crib.
- Use "tummy time" when awake.
- Learn baby's responses, temperament, likes/dislikes.
- Develop strategies for fussy times.
  How much is your baby crying? What are some ways you have found to calm your baby? What do you do if that doesn't work?

INFANT-FAMILY SYNCHRONY

Parent-infant separation (return to work/school), child care

- Plan for return to school/work.
- Choose quality child care; recognize that separation is hard.
  How do you feel about leaving your baby with someone else?

NUTRITIONAL ADEQUACY

Feeding routine, feeding choices (delaying complementary foods, herbs/vitamins/supplements), hunger/satiation cues, feeding strategies (holding, burping), feeding guidance (breastfeeding, formula)

- Exclusive breastfeeding during the first 4-6 months is ideal; iron-fortified formula is recommended substitute; recognize signs of hunger, fullness; burp at natural breaks; no extra fluids or food.
- *If breastfeeding:* Continue with 8-12 feedings in 24 hours; plan for pumping/storing breast milk if returning to work/school.
- *If formula feeding:* Prepare/store formula safely; feed every 3-4 hours; hold baby semi-upright; don't prop bottle; no bottle in bed.

SAFETY

Car safety seats, water temperature (hot liquids), choking, tobacco smoke, drowning, falls (rolling over)

- Use rear-facing car safety seat in back seat; never put baby in front seat of vehicle with passenger air bag.
- Always use safety belt; do not drive under the influence of alcohol or drugs.
- Don't drink hot liquids while holding baby; set home water temperature <120°F.
- Don't smoke; keep home/vehicle smoke-free.
- Don't leave baby alone in tub or high places (changing tables, beds, sofas); keep hand on baby.
- Keep small objects, plastic bags away from baby.

Observation of Parent-Child Interaction: Are parents and infant responsive to each other? Do parents comfort when infant cries? Are parents attentive to infant? Do parents and infant demonstrate reciprocal engagement around feeding/eating? Do parents respond to infant's cues and how does the infant respond?

Surveillance of Development: Smiles spontaneously, elicits social interactions, shows solidified self-consolation skills; cries in differentiated manner, babbles expressively and spontaneously; responds to affection/changes in environment, indicates pleasure/displeasure; pushes chest to elbows, has good head control, demonstrates symmetrical movements of arms/legs, begins to roll and reach for objects.

Physical Exam. Complete, including: Measure and plot length, weight, head circumference. Plot weight-for-length. Assess/Observe rashes, bruising; positional skull deformities; ocular mobility for lateral gaze, pupil opacification, red reflexes. Ascult for heart murmurs. Palpate femoral pulses. Assess/Observe developmental hip dysplasia; neurologic tone, strength, and movement symmetry.

Screening (See p 58.)

Universal: None
Selective: Blood Pressure; Vision; Hearing; Anemia

Immunizations

DC: www.cdc.gov/vaccines
AAP: www.aapredbook.org

Anticipatory Guidance

FAMILY FUNCTIONING

Parent roles/responsibilities, parental responses to infant, child care providers (number, quality)

- Take time for self, partner; maintain social contacts; spend time with your other children.
- Hold, cuddle, talk/sing to baby.
- Learn baby's responses, temperament, likes/dislikes.

What do you think your baby is trying to tell you when she cries, looks at you, turns away, smiles?

- Make quality child care arrangements.

INFANT DEVELOPMENT

Consistent daily routines, sleep (crib safety, sleep location), parent-child relationship (play, tummy time), infant self-regulation (social development, infant self-calming)

- Continue regular feeding/sleeping routines; put baby to bed awake but drowsy.

12

Key= Guidance for parents, *questions*

- Put baby to sleep on back; don't use loose, soft bedding; lower crib mattress before baby can sit up; choose mesh playpen with weave $<\frac{1}{4}$"; never leave baby in with drop side down.
- Use quiet (reading, singing) and active ("tummy time") playtime; provide safe opportunities to explore.
- Continue calming strategies when fussy.
  What do you do to calm your baby? Do you ever feel that you or other caretakers may hurt the baby? How do you handle that feeling?

NUTRITION ADEQUACY AND GROWTH

Feeding success, weight gain, feeding choices (complementary foods, food allergies), feeding guidance (breastfeeding, formula)

- Exclusive breastfeeding during the first 4-6 months is ideal; iron-fortified formula is recommended substitute.
- Cereal can be introduced between 4-6 months, when child is developmentally ready.
- *If breastfeeding:* Recognize growth spurts; plan for safe pumping/storing of breast milk.
- *If formula feeding:* Prepare/store formula safely; 8 to 12 times in 24 hours; hold baby semi-upright; don't prop bottle; no bottle in bed; consider contacting WIC.

ORAL HEALTH

Maternal oral health care, use of clean pacifier, teething/drooling, avoidance of bottle in bed

- Don't share spoon or clean pacifier in your mouth; maintain good dental hygiene.
- Avoid bottle in bed, propping, "grazing."

SAFETY

Car safety seats, falls, walkers, lead poisoning, drowning, water temperature (hot liquids), burns, choking

- Use rear-facing car safety seat in back seat; never put baby in front seat of vehicle with passenger air bag.
- Always use safety belt; do not drive under the influence of alcohol or drugs.
- Don't leave baby alone in tub, high places (changing tables, beds, sofas); keep hand on baby; don't use infant walker.
- Set home water temperature <120°F.
- Avoid burn risk to baby (hot liquids, cooking, ironing, smoking).
- Keep small objects, plastic bags away from baby.
- Check for sources of lead in home.

Observation of Parent-Child Interaction: Are the parents and infant responsive to one another? Do the parents show confidence with infant? Does the parent-infant relationship demonstrate comfort, adequate feeding/eating, and response to the infant's cues? Do parents/partners support each other?

Surveillance of Development: Is socially interactive with parent, recognizes familiar faces, babbles, enjoys vocal turn taking, starts to know own name; uses visual and oral exploration to learn about environment; rolls over and sits, stands and bounces; moves to crawling from prone; rocks back and forth; is learning to rotate in sitting; will move from sitting to crawling.

Physical Exam. Complete, including: Measure and plot length, weight, head circumference. Plot weight-for-length. Assess/Observe rashes, bruising; ocular mobility, eye alignment, pupil opacification, red reflexes. Ascult for heart murmurs. Palpate femoral pulses. Assess/Observe developmental hip dysplasia, neurologic tone, movement strength and symmetry.

Screening (See p 58.)

Universal: Oral Health
Selective: Blood Pressure; Vision; Hearing; Lead; Tuberculosis

Immunizations

CDC: www.cdc.gov/vaccines
AAP: www.aapredbook.org

Anticipatory Guidance

FAMILY FUNCTIONING

Balancing parent roles (health care decision making, parent support systems), child care

- Use support networks.
  How are you balancing your roles of partner and parent? Who are you able to go to when you need help with your family?
- Choose responsible, trusted child care providers; consider playgroups.

Key= Guidance for parents, *questions*

INFANT DEVELOPMENT

Parent expectations (parents as teachers), infant developmental changes (cognitive development/learning, playtime), communication (babbling, reciprocal activities, early intervention), emerging infant independence (infant self-regulation/behavior management), sleep routine (self-calming/putting self to sleep, crib safety)

- Use high chair/upright seat so baby can see you.

- Engage in interactive, reciprocal play. Talk/sing to, read/play games with baby.

  How does your baby communicate or tell you what he wants and needs?

- Continue regular daily routines; put baby to bed awake but drowsy.
- Put baby to sleep on back; choose crib with slats $\leq 2\frac{3}{8}$" apart; don't use loose, soft bedding; lower crib mattress; choose mesh playpen with weave $<\frac{1}{4}$"; never leave baby in with drop side down.

NUTRITION AND FEEDING: ADEQUACY/GROWTH

Feeding strategies (quantity, limits, location, responsibilities), feeding choices (complementary foods, choices of fluids/juice), feeding guidance (breastfeeding, formula)

- Exclusive breastfeeding during the first 4-6 months is ideal; iron-fortified formula is recommended substitute; recognize slowing rate of growth.
- Determine whether baby is ready for solids; introduce single-ingredient foods one at a time; provide iron-rich foods; respond to baby's cues.
- Begin cup; limit juice (2-4 oz a day).
- *If breastfeeding:* Continue as long as mutually desired.
- *If formula feeding:* Don't switch to milk; contact WIC/community resources for help.

ORAL HEALTH

Fluoride, oral hygiene/soft toothbrush, avoidance of bottle in bed

- Assess fluoride source.
- Brush with soft toothbrush/cloth and water.
- Avoid bottle in bed, propping, "grazing."

SAFETY

Car safety seats, burns (hot water/hot surfaces), falls (gates at stairs and no walkers), choking, poisoning, drowning

- Use rear-facing car safety seat in back seat until 1 year AND 20 pounds; never put in front seat of vehicle with passenger air bag.
- Do home safety check (stair gates, barriers around space heaters, cleaning products).
- Don't leave baby alone in tub, high places (changing tables, beds, sofas); don't use infant walker.
- Keep baby in high chair/playpen when in kitchen.
- Set home water temperature <120°F.
- Avoid burn risk to baby (stoves, heaters).
- Keep small objects, plastic bags, away from baby.
- To prevent choking, limit "finger foods" to soft bits.

15

Observation of Parent-Child Interaction: Do parents stimulate the infant with language, play? Do parents and infant demonstrate reciprocal engagement around feeding/eating? Can infant move away from parent to explore and check back with parent visually and physically? Are parents' developmental expectations appropriate? How do parents respond to infant's independent behavior within a safe environment?

Surveillance of Development: Has developed apprehension with strangers, seeks out parent; uses repetitive consonants and vowel sounds, points out objects; develops object permanence, learns interactive games, explores environment; expands motor skills.

Physical Exam. Complete, including: Measure and plot length, weight, head circumference. Plot weight-for-length. Assess/Observe positional skull deformities; ocular mobility, eye alignment, pupil opacification, red reflexes. Ascult for heart murmurs. Palpate femoral pulses. Assess/Observe developmental hip dysplasia; neurologic tone, movement strength and symmetry. Elicit parachute reflex.

Screening (See p 58.)

Universal: Development; Oral Health
Selective: Blood Pressure; Vision; Hearing; Lead

Immunizations

CDC: www.cdc.gov/vaccines
AAP: www.aapredbook.org

Anticipatory Guidance

FAMILY ADAPTATIONS

Discipline (parenting expectations, consistency, behavior management), cultural beliefs about child-rearing, family functioning, domestic violence

• Use consistent, positive discipline (limit use of the word "No," use distraction, be a role model).

• Make time for self, partner, friends.
• Ask for help with domestic violence.
  Do you always feel safe in your home? Has your partner or ex-partner ever hit you? Are you scared that you or other caretakers may hurt the baby? Would you like information on where to go and who to contact for help?

16

Key= Guidance for parents, *questions*

INFANT INDEPENDENCE

Changing sleep pattern (sleep schedule), developmental mobility (safe exploration, play), cognitive development (object permanence, separation anxiety, behavior and learning, temperament versus self-regulation, visual exploration, cause and effect), communication

- Keep consistent daily routines.
- Provide opportunities for safe exploration, be realistic about abilities.
  How does your baby adapt to new situations, people, and places?
- Recognize new social skills, separation anxiety; be sensitive to temperament.
- Play with cause-and-effect toys; talk/sing/read together; respond to baby's cues.
  How do you think the baby is learning? How is he communicating with you?
- Avoid TV, videos, computers.

FEEDING ROUTINE

Self-feeding, mealtime routines, transition to solids (table-food introduction), cup drinking (plans for weaning)

- Gradually increase table foods; ensure variety of foods, textures.
- Provide 3 meals, 2-3 snacks a day.
- Encourage use of cup; discuss plans for weaning.
- Continue breastfeeding if mutually desired.

SAFETY

Car safety seats, burns (hot stoves, heaters), window guards, drowning, poisoning (safety locks), guns

- Use rear-facing car safety seat in back seat until 1 year AND 20 pounds; never put baby in front seat of vehicle with passenger air bag.
- Always use safety belt; do not drive under the influence of alcohol or drugs.
- Don't leave heavy objects, hot liquids on tablecloths.
- Do home safety check (stair gates, barriers around space heaters, cleaning products, electrical cords).
- Keep baby in high chair/playpen when in kitchen.
- Install operable window guards on second- and higher-story windows.
- Be within arm's reach ("touch supervision") near water, pools, bathtubs.
- Put Poison Control Center number at each telephone.

17

Observation of Parent-Child Interaction: How does parent interact with toddler? Does child check back with parent visually? Does toddler bring an object to show parent? How does parent react to praise of self or child by health care professional? How do siblings interact with toddler? Does parent seem positive about child?

Surveillance of Development: Plays interactive games, imitates activities, hands parent a book when wants a story, waves "bye-bye," has strong attachment with parent and shows distress on separation; demonstrates protodeclarative pointing; imitates vocalizations/sounds; speaks 1-2 words; jabbers with normal inflections; follows simple directions, identifies people upon request; bangs 2 cubes held in hands, stands alone.

Physical Exam. Complete, including: Measure and plot length, weight, head circumference. Plot weight-for-length. Examine for red reflexes. Perform cover/uncover test. Observe for caries, plaque, demineralization, staining. Observe gait. Determine whether testes fully descended.

Screening (See p 59.)

Universal: Anemia; Lead (high prevalence/Medicaid)
Selective: Oral Health; Blood Pressure; Vision; Hearing; Lead (low prevalence/no Medicaid); Tuberculosis

Immunizations

CDC: www.cdc.gov/vaccines
AAP: www.aapredbook.org

Anticipatory Guidance

FAMILY SUPPORT

Adjustment to the child's developmental changes and behavior, family-work balance, parental agreement/disagreement about child issues

- Discipline with time-outs and positive distractions; praise for good behaviors.
  When your child is troublesome, what do you do?

- Make time for self and partner; time with family; keep ties with friends.
- Maintain or expand ties to your community; consider parent-toddler playgroups, parent education, or support group.
  Who do you talk to about parenting issues?

18

Key= Guidance for parent, *questions*

ESTABLISHING ROUTINES

Family time, bedtime, teeth brushing, nap times

- Establish family traditions.
  What do you all do together? Tell me about your family's traditions.
- Continue 1 nap a day; nightly bedtime routine with quiet time, reading, singing, a favorite toy.
- Establish teeth brushing routine.

FEEDING AND APPETITE CHANGES

Self-feeding, nutritious foods, choices, "grazing"

- Encourage self-feeding; avoid small, hard foods.
- Feed 3 meals and 2-3 nutritious snacks a day; be sure caregivers do the same.
- Provide nutritious food and healthy snacks.
- Trust child to decide how much to eat (toddlers tend to "graze").

ESTABLISHING A DENTAL HOME

First dental checkup, dental hygiene

- Visit the dentist by 12 months or after first tooth.
- Brush teeth twice a day with plain water, soft toothbrush.
- If still using bottle, offer only water.

SAFETY

Home safety, car safety seats, drowning, guns

- "Childproof" home (medications, cleaning supplies, heaters, dangling cords, stairs, small or sharp objects).
- Use a rear-facing car safety seat until at least 1 year old AND at least 20 pounds.
- It is best to use a rear-facing car safety seat until highest weight or height allowed by manufacturer; make necessary changes when switching to forward facing; never place rear-facing car safety seat in front seat of vehicle with passenger air bag; back seat is safest.
- Stay within an arm's reach ("touch supervision") when near water; empty buckets, pools, bathtubs immediately after use.
- Remove guns from home; if gun necessary, store unloaded and locked, with ammunition locked separately.

Observation of Parent-Child Interaction: What is the emotional tone between parent and child? How does parent support toddler's need for safety and reassurance in exam? Does toddler check back with parent visually? How does parent react to praise from health care professional? How do siblings react to toddler?

Surveillance of Development: Listens to a story, imitates activities, may help in house; indicates wants by pulling/pointing/grunting, brings objects to show, hands a book when wants a story; says 2-3 words with meaning; understands/follows simple commands, scribbles; walks well, stoops, recovers, can step backwards; puts block in cup, drinks from cup.

Physical Exam. Complete, including: Measure and plot length, weight, head circumference. Plot weight-for-length. Examine red reflexes. Perform cover/uncover test. Observe for caries, plaque, demineralization, staining. Observe for stranger avoidance.

Screening (See p 59.)

Universal: None
Selective: Blood Pressure; Vision; Hearing

Immunizations

CDC: www.cdc.gov/vaccines
AAP: www.aapredbook.org

Anticipatory Guidance

COMMUNICATION AND SOCIAL DEVELOPMENT

Individuation, separation, attention to how child communicates wants and interests, signs of shared attention

- When possible, allow child to choose between 2 options acceptable to you.
- "Stranger anxiety" and separation anxiety reflect new cognitive gains; speak reassuringly.
- Use simple, clear words and phrases to promote language development and improve communication.

How does your child communicate what she wants? Does she point to something she wants and then watch to see if you see what she's doing?

SLEEP ROUTINES AND ISSUES

Regular bedtime routine, night waking, no bottle in bed

- Maintain consistent bedtime and nighttime routine; tuck in when drowsy, but still awake.
- If night waking occurs, reassure briefly, give stuffed animal or blanket for self-consolation.
- Do not give bottle in bed.

Key= Guidance for parent, *questions*

TEMPER TANTRUMS AND DISCIPLINE

Conflict predictors, distraction, praise for accomplishments, consistency

- Some conflict/tantrums can be avoided by "toddler-proofing" home, using distractions, accepting messiness, allowing child to choose (when appropriate).
  What kinds of things do you find yourself saying "No" about?
- Praise good behavior and accomplishments.
- Use discipline for teaching/protecting, not punishing.
  How are you and your partner managing your child's behavior? What do you do when you disagree?

HEALTHY TEETH

Brushing teeth, bottle usage

- Schedule first dental visit if hasn't seen dentist yet.
- Brush teeth twice a day with soft brush and plain water.
- Prevent tooth decay by good family oral health habits (brushing, flossing), not sharing utensils or cup.
- If nighttime bottle, use water only.

SAFETY

Car safety seats, parental use of safety belts, poison, fire safety

- It is best to use rear-facing car safety seat until highest weight or height allowed by manufacturer; make necessary changes when switching a convertible seat to forward facing; never place rear-facing car safety seat in front seat of vehicle with passenger air bag; back seat is safest.
- Make sure everyone uses a safety belt.
- Review home safety (remove or lock up poisons, cleaning supplies; use stair gates; install operable window guards on second- and higher-story windows).
  When did you last examine your home to make sure it is safe? What emergency numbers do you have posted near your phones?
- Install smoke detector on every level, test monthly/change batteries annually; make fire escape plan; set hot water <120°F.
- Keep hot liquids, lighters, matches out of reach.

21

Observation of Parent-Child Interaction: How do the parent and child communicate? Does child show parent book? Does parent ask child many questions or give many directions? What is the tone of parent-child interactions? How does parent guide child to safe limits?

Surveillance of Development: Is interactive/withdrawn, friendly/aggressive; laughs in response to others, explores alone but with parent nearby; vocalizes and gestures, speaks 6 words, points to indicate wants; points to 1 body part, follows simple instructions, knows names of favorite books; walks up steps/runs; stacks 2 or 3 blocks, scribbles, uses spoon/cup without spilling.

Physical Exam. Complete, including: Measure and plot recumbent length, weight, head circumference. Plot weight-for-length. Observe gait, hand control, arm/spine movement. Examine for red reflexes. Perform cover/uncover test. Observe for nevi, café au lait spots, birthmarks, bruising; caries, plaque, demineralization, staining, injury.

Screening (See p 59.)

Universal: Development, Autism
Selective: Oral Health, Blood Pressure, Vision, Hearing, Anemia, Lead, Tuberculosis

Immunizations

CDC: www.cdc.gov/vaccines
AAP: www.aapredbook.org

Anticipatory Guidance

FAMILY SUPPORT

Parental well-being, adjustment to toddler's growing independence and occasional negativity, queries about a new sibling planned or on the way

- Create family times; spend time with each child; take actions to ensure own health.
  What activities do you do as a family? Tell me if you have ever been in a relationship where you have been hurt, threatened, or treated badly? What did you do?
- Support emerging independence but reinforce limits and appropriate behavior.
- Prepare toddler for new sibling by reading books together about a new baby.

22

Key= Guidance for parent, *questions*

CHILD DEVELOPMENT AND BEHAVIOR

Adaptation to nonparental care and anticipation of return to clinging, other changes connected with new cognitive gains

- Anticipate anxiety/clinging in new situations.
- Praise good behavior/accomplishments.
- Be consistent with discipline/enforcing limits, share with other caregivers.
- Enjoy daily playtime.

LANGUAGE PROMOTION/HEARING

Encouragement of language, use of simple words/phrases, engagement in reading/singing/talking

- Encourage language development by reading and singing; talk about what you see.
- Use simple words to describe pictures in book.
- Use words that describe feelings and emotions to help child learn about feelings.
  How does your child communicate what she wants?

TOILET TRAINING READINESS

Recognizing signs of readiness, parental expectations

- Wait until child is ready (dry for periods of about 2 hours, knows wet and dry, can pull pants up/down, can indicate bowel movement).
- Read books about using the potty, praise attempts to sit on the potty.

SAFETY

Car safety seats; parental use of safety belts; falls, fires, and burns; poisoning; guns

- It is best to use a rear-facing car safety seat until highest weight or height allowed by manufacturer; make necessary changes when switching a convertible seat to forward facing; never place rear-facing car safety seat in front seat of vehicle with passenger air bag; back seat is safest.
- Make sure everyone uses a safety belt.
- Use stair gates, install operable window guards on second- and higher-story windows.
- Prevent burns (hot liquids/stove/matches/lighters). Install smoke detectors.
- Remove guns from home; if gun necessary, store unloaded and locked, with ammunition locked separately.

Note: Bright Futures recommends anticipatory guidance on reading aloud at every visit from 6 months to 5 years and encourages giving a book at these visits. For more information, visit www.reachoutandread.org.

23

Observation of Parent-Child Interaction: How do parent and child communicate? What is tone of the interaction and the feelings conveyed? Does child feel free to explore the room? How does the parent set limits?

Surveillance of Development: Imitates adults, plays alongside other children, refers to self as "I" or "me," has at least 50 words, uses 2-word phrases, asks parent to read a book; follows 2-step commands, completes sentences and rhymes in familiar books; stacks 5 or 6 blocks, makes or imitates horizontal and circular strokes with crayon, turns pages one at a time, imitates food preparation, throws ball overhand; goes up and down stairs one step at a time, jumps up.

Physical Exam. Complete, including: Measure standing height (preferred) or recumbent length, weight, head circumference. Calculate and plot BMI, or plot weight-for-length. Examine for red reflexes. Perform cover/uncover test. Observe for caries, plaque, demineralization, staining, injury, gingivitis. Observe running, scribbling, socialization, ability to follow commands. Assess language acquisition/clarity.

Screening (See p 59.)

Universal: Autism; Lead (high prevalence/Medicaid)
Selective: Oral Health; Blood Pressure; Vision; Hearing; Anemia; Lead (low prevalence/no Medicaid); Tuberculosis; Dyslipidemia

Immunizations

CDC: www.cdc.gov/vaccines
AAP: www.aapredbook.org

Anticipatory Guidance

ASSESSMENT OF LANGUAGE DEVELOPMENT

How child communicates, expectations for language

- Model appropriate language.
- Read together every day; child may love same story over and over.
- Recognize that child may struggle to respond quickly; talk and question slowly.
- Should be able to follow simple 1 or 2 step commands.
  What do you think your child understands?

Key= Guidance for parent, *questions*

TEMPERAMENT AND BEHAVIOR

Sensitivity, approachability, adaptability, intensity

- Praise good behavior/accomplishments; listen to and respect your child.
- Help child express such feelings as joy, anger, sadness, frustration.
- Encourage self-expression.
  Tell me about your child's typical play.
- Learn child's way of reacting to people/situations.
- Encourage child to play with other children.
  How does your child act around other children?

TOILET TRAINING

What have parents tried, techniques, personal hygiene

- Begin when child is ready (dry for periods of 2 hours, knows wet and dry, can pull pants up/down, can indicate bowel movement).
- Plan for frequent toilet breaks (up to 10 times a day).
- Teach personal hygiene (wash hands, sneeze/cough into shoulder).

TELEVISION VIEWING

Limits on viewing, promotion of reading, promotion of physical activity and safe play

- Limit TV and video to no more than 1-2 hours of quality programming per day.
- If you allow TV, watch together and discuss.
- Choose TV alternatives (reading, games, singing).
- Encourage physical activity; be active as a family.

SAFETY

Car safety seats, parental use of safety belts, bike helmets, outdoor safety, guns

- Install car safety seat in back seat.
- Make sure everyone else uses a safety belt.
- Use bike helmet.
- Supervise child outside, especially around cars, machinery, in streets.
- Remove guns from home; if gun necessary, store unloaded and locked, with ammunition locked separately.

Observation of Parent-Child Interaction: How actively do parent and child communicate? Does the child use questions and phrases at appropriate age level? Do parent and child look at book, discuss, and interact? How well does parent calm child?

Surveillance of Development: Play includes other children; has fears about unexplained changes in environment/unexpected events; uses phrases of 3-4 words, is understandable to others 50% of the time; knows the correct action for animal or person (eg, bird flies, man talks), points to 6 body parts; jumps up and down in place, throws ball overhand, brushes teeth with help, puts on clothes with help, copies vertical line.

Physical Exam. Complete, including: Measure and plot standing height (preferred) or recumbent length, weight, head circumference. Calculate and plot BMI, or plot weight-for-length. Examine red reflexes. Perform cover/uncover test. Observe coordination, language acquisition/clarity, socialization. Assess vocalizations.

Screening (See p 59.)

Universal: Development
Selective: Oral Health; Blood Pressure; Vision; Hearing

Immunizations

CDC: www.cdc.gov/vaccines
AAP: www.aapredbook.org

Anticipatory Guidance

FAMILY ROUTINES

Parental consistency, day and evening routines, enjoyable family activities

• Reach agreement with all family members on how best to support child's emerging independence while maintaining consistent limits.
How well do you and your family agree on limits and discipline for your child?

• Encourage family exercise (walking, swimming, biking).
Tell me how you have fun with your family.
• Maintain regular family routines (meals, daily reading).

LANGUAGE PROMOTION AND COMMUNICATION

Interactive communication through song, play, and reading

• Read together every day; go to the library.
Does he enjoy having stories read to him? Does he enjoy songs, rhymes, and games with you?
• Limit TV and video to no more than 1-2 hours a day; monitor what child watches.

26

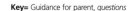

- Listen when child speaks; repeat, using correct grammar.
  Is your child speaking in sentences?

PROMOTING SOCIAL DEVELOPMENT

Play with other children, limited reciprocal play, imitation of others, choices

- Encourage play with other children, but supervise because child not ready yet to share/play cooperatively.
- Build independence by offering choices between 2 acceptable alternatives.
  Does your child enjoy making independent decisions? What are some of the new things your child is doing?

PRESCHOOL CONSIDERATIONS

Readiness for early childhood programs, playgroups, or playdates

- Consider group child care, preschool program, organized playdates or playgroups.
  What are your plans for child care or preschool in the year ahead?
- Encourage toilet-training success by dressing child in easy-to-remove clothes, establish daily routine, place on potty every 1-2 hours, praise, maintain relaxed environment by reading/singing.

SAFETY

Water safety, car safety seats, outdoor health and safety (pools, play areas, sun exposure), pets, fires and burns

- Stay within an arm's reach ("touch supervision") near water, bathtubs, pools, toilet.
- Properly install car safety seat in back seat.
- Supervise child outside, especially around cars, machinery; use bike helmet; limit sun, use sunscreen.
- Install smoke detectors on every level, test monthly and change batteries annually; make fire escape plan; keep matches out of sight.

Observation of Parent-Child Interaction: How do parent and child communicate? Does parent give child choices? Does parent encourage the child's cooperation? Does unacceptable behavior elicit appropriate responses?

Surveillance of Development: Has self-care skills (eg, feeding, dressing); imaginative play becomes more elaborate, enjoys interactive play; converses in 2-3 sentences, understandable to others 75% of the time, names a friend; knows name, identifies self as girl/boy; builds tower of 6-8 cubes, throws ball overhand, walks up stairs alternating feet; copies a circle, draws person with 2 body parts; day toilet trained for bowel and bladder.

Physical Exam. Complete, including: Measure blood pressure. Measure and plot height, weight. Calculate and plot BMI. Attempt ophthalmoscopic exam of optic nerve and retinal vessels. Observe for caries, plaque, demineralization, staining, injury, gingivitis; language acquisition, speech clarity; adult-child interaction.

Screening (See p 59.)

Universal: Visual Acuity
Selective: Oral Health; Hearing; Anemia; Lead; Tuberculosis

Immunizations

CDC: www.cdc.gov/vaccines
AAP: www.aapredbook.org

Anticipatory Guidance

FAMILY SUPPORT

Family decisions, sibling rivalry, work balance

- Be aware of differences/similarities in your parenting style and that of your parents.
- Show affection; handle anger constructively; reinforce limits/appropriate behavior.

Tell me how family members show affection, anger? Describe what your family does together.
- Help children develop good relations with each other; spend time with each child.
  How do your children get along together?
  What do you like to do best with your brothers and sisters?
- Take time for yourself; spend time alone with your partner.

Key= Guidance for parent, *questions;* Guidance for child, *questions*

ENCOURAGING LITERACY ACTIVITIES

Singing, talking, describing, observing, reading

- Read, sing, play rhyme games together.
- Talk about pictures in books (don't always have to read); let child "tell" story.
- Encourage child to talk about friends, experiences.
  How does your child tell you what he wants? How well does the family understand his speech?

PLAYING WITH PEERS

Interactive games, play opportunities

- Encourage play with appropriate toys and safe exploration; fantasy play.
  Tell me about your child's typical play.
- Encourage interactive games with peers; taking turns.

PROMOTING PHYSICAL ACTIVITY

Limits on inactivity

- Create opportunities for family to share time and exercise together.
- Promote daily physical activity at home, in child care or in preschool.
- Limit all screen time to no more than 1-2 hours a day; no TV/DVD player in bedroom; monitor programs watched.

SAFETY

Car safety seats, pedestrian safety, falls from windows, guns

- Use forward-facing car safety seat, properly installed in back seat.
- Switch to belt-positioning booster seat when child reaches highest weight/height allowed by manufacturer of forward-facing seat with harness.
- Supervise all play near streets/driveways; do not allow child to cross street alone.
- Move furniture away from windows; install operable window guards on second- and higher-story windows.
- Remove guns from home; if gun necessary, store unloaded and locked, with ammunition locked separately; ask if guns in home where child plays.

Observation of Parent-Child Interaction: How do parent and child communicate? Does parent allow child to answer questions? Does child separate from parent during exam? Does child dress and undress self? How do parent, child, siblings interact? If offered books, does parent let child choose?

Surveillance of Development: Describes features of self; listens to stories, engages in fantasy play; gives first/last name, knows what to do if cold/tired/hungry, most speech clearly understandable; names 4 colors, plays board/card games, draws a person with 3 parts; hops on one foot, balances on one foot for 2 seconds, builds tower of 8 blocks, copies a cross; brushes own teeth, dresses self.

Physical Exam. Complete, including: Measure blood pressure. Measure and plot height, weight. Calculate and plot BMI. Observe fine/gross motor skills. Assess language acquisition, speech fluency/clarity, thought content/abstraction.

Screening (See p 59.)

Universal: Visual Acuity; Hearing
Selective: Anemia; Lead; Tuberculosis; Dyslipidemia

Immunizations

CDC: www.cdc.gov/vaccines
AAP: www.aapredbook.org

Anticipatory Guidance

SCHOOL READINESS

Structured learning experiences, opportunities to socialize with other children, fears, friends, fluency

• Children are very sensitive, easily encouraged or hurt; model respectful behavior and apologize if wrong; praise when demonstrates sensitivity to feelings of others.

• Provide opportunities to play with other children.
  How interested is your child in other children? How confident is she socially and emotionally?
  Do you have a favorite friend?

• Consider structured learning (preschool, Head Start, or community program); visit parks, museums, libraries.
  How happy are you with your child care arrangements? Does she seem happy to go?

• Reading is important to help child like reading and be ready for school.

30

Key= Guidance for parent, *questions;* Guidance for child, *questions*

- Give child time to finish sentences; encourage speaking skills by reading/talking together.
  How does your child communicate what she wants and knows?

DEVELOPING HEALTHY PERSONAL HABITS
Daily routines that promote health

- Create calm bedtime ritual, mealtimes without TV, toothbrushing twice a day with pea-sized toothpaste.

TELEVISION/MEDIA
Limits on viewing, promotion of physical activity and safe play

- Limit TV and video to 1-2 hours a day; no TV in bedroom; watch programs together and discuss.
- Make opportunities for daily play; be physically active as a family.

CHILD AND FAMILY INVOLVEMENT AND SAFETY IN THE COMMUNITY
Activities outside the home, community projects, educational programs, relating to peers and adults, domestic violence

- Maintain or expand participation in community activities.
- Expect curiosity about the body; use correct terms, answer questions.
- Teach your child rules for how to be safe with adults, using 3 principles: (1) no adult should tell a child to keep secrets from parents, (2) no adult should express interest in private parts, (3) no adult should ask a child for help with his/her private parts.
- Know that help is available if personal safety is a concern.
  Many children I see have parents who have been hurt by someone else, so I ask about it routinely. Are you scared that your partner or someone else may try to hurt you or your child?

SAFETY
Belt-positioning booster seats, supervision, outdoor safety, guns

- Use a forward-facing car safety seat installed in back seat until child reaches highest weight or height allowed by manufacturer of forward-facing seat with harness. Then switch to belt-positioning booster seat.
  Where do you sit when you ride in the car? Do you have a special seat?
- Supervise all outdoor play, never leave child alone outside; do not allow child to cross street alone.
- Remove guns from home; if gun necessary, store unloaded and locked, with ammunition locked separately. Ask if guns are in homes where child plays.

Observation of Parent-Child Interaction: How do parent and child interact with health care professional? How do parent and child interact? Does parent have realistic expectations about child?

Surveillance of Development: Balances on one foot, hops, and skips; able to tie a knot. Shows school readiness skills: has mature pencil grasp, can draw a person with at least 6 body parts, prints some letters and numbers, is able to copy squares and triangles, has good articulation/language skills, counts to 10, names 4+ colors, follows simple directions, listens and attends.

Physical Exam. Complete, including: Measure blood pressure. Measure and plot height, weight. Calculate and plot BMI. Attempt ophthalmoscopic exam of optic nerve and retinal vessels. Observe for caries, gingival inflammation, malocclusion; fine/gross motor skills; gait. Assess language acquisition, speech fluency/clarity, thought content, ability to understand abstract thinking.

Screening (See p 60.)

5 Year Visit
Universal: Vision; Hearing
Selective: Anemia; Lead; Tuberculosis

6 Year Visit
Universal: Vision; Hearing
Selective: Oral Health; Anemia; Lead; Tuberculosis; Dyslipidemia

Immunizations

CDC: www.cdc.gov/vaccines
AAP: www.aapredbook.org

Anticipatory Guidance

SCHOOL READINESS

Established routines, after-school care and activities, parent-teacher communication, friends, bullying, maturity, management of disappointments, fears

- Prepare child for school; tour school; attend back-to-school events.
  What concerns do you have about your child's ability to do well in school?
- Be sure after-school care is safe, positive.
- Talk to child about school experiences.
- Talk to parents about school, worries.
  Tell me about your new school. Do kids ever call you mean names or tease you?

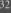

Key= Guidance for parent, *questions;* Guidance for child, *questions*

MENTAL HEALTH

Family time, routines, temper problems, social interactions

- Continue family routines; assign household chores.
- Show affection/respect; model anger management/self-discipline.
- Use discipline for teaching, not punishing.
- Solve conflict/anger by talking, going outside and playing, walking away.
  What makes you sad, angry? How do you handle it?

NUTRITION AND PHYSICAL ACTIVITY

Healthy weight; appropriate well-balanced diet; increased fruit, vegetable, whole-grain consumption; adequate calcium intake; 60 minutes of exercise a day

- Eat breakfast; eat 5+ servings of fruits/vegetables a day.
- Limit candy/soda/high-fat snacks.
- Have at least 2 cups low-fat milk/other dairy a day.
- Be physically active 60 minutes a day.
- Limit TV to 2 hours a day; no TV in bedroom.

ORAL HEALTH

Regular visits with dentist, daily brushing and flossing, adequate fluoride

- Help child with brushing if needed.
- Visit dentist twice a year.
- Give fluoride supplement if dentist recommends.
- Brush teeth twice a day; floss once.

SAFETY

Pedestrian safety, booster seat, safety helmets, swimming safety, child sexual abuse prevention, fire escape/drill plan and smoke detectors, carbon monoxide detectors/alarms, guns

- Teach safe street habits (crossing/riding school bus).
- Use properly positioned belt-positioning booster seat in back seat.
- Ensure child uses safety equipment (helmet, pads).
- Teach child to swim; supervise around water; use sunscreen.
- Teach rules for how to be safe with adults: (1) no adult should tell a child to keep secrets from parents, (2) no adult should express interest in private parts, (3) no adult should ask a child for help with his/her private parts; explain "privates."
  Have you talked to your child about ways to avoid sexual abuse? What would you do if a grown-up made you scared? Who could you tell? Who would help you?
- Install smoke detectors/carbon monoxide detector/alarms; make fire escape plan.
- Remove guns from home; if gun necessary, store unloaded and locked with ammunition locked separately.

Observation of Parent-Child Interaction: How do parent and child interact? Does parent have realistic expectations about child? How does child interact with adults other than parents?

Surveillance of Development:
- Physical, cognitive, emotional, social, moral competencies
- Caring, supportive relationship with family, other adults, peers

Physical Exam. Complete, including: Measure blood pressure. Measure and plot height, weight. Calculate and plot BMI. Observe hip/knee/ankle function. Observe for caries, gingival inflammation, and malocclusion. Assess for SMR.

Screening (See p 60.)

7 Year Visit
Universal: None
Selective: Vision; Hearing; Anemia; Tuberculosis

8 Year Visit
Universal: Vision; Hearing
Selective: Anemia; Tuberculosis; Dyslipidemia

Immunizations

CDC: www.cdc.gov/vaccines
AAP: www.aapredbook.org

Key= Guidance for parent, *questions;* Guidance for child, *questions*

Anticipatory Guidance

SCHOOL

Adaptation to school, school problems (behavior or learning issues), school performance/progress, involvement in school activities and after-school programs, bullying, parental involvement, IEP or special education services

- Show interest in school and activities.
  How is your child doing in school? How do you help your child solve conflicts?

  How do you like school? Are you picked on by others?
- If concerns, ask teacher about evaluation for special help/tutoring; help with bullying.

DEVELOPMENT AND MENTAL HEALTH

Independence, self-esteem, establishing rules and consequences, temper problems, managing and resolving conflicts, puberty/pubertal development

- Encourage competence/independence.
  What new things have you tried recently?
- Show affection, praise child.
- Be positive role model; do not hit or let others hit.
- Discuss rules, consequences.
  What types of discipline do you use most often?
- Talk about worries.
  Who do you talk to about your worries and things that make you mad?

- Be aware of pubertal changes; answer questions simply.
  What have you told your child about how to care for his changing body?

  Do you know what puberty is? Has anyone talked with you about how your body will change during puberty?

NUTRITION AND PHYSICAL ACTIVITY

Healthy weight, appropriate food intake, adequate calcium, water instead of soda, adequate physical activity in organized sports/after-school programs/fun activities, limits on screen time

- Encourage nutritious food choices.
  What do you think of your child's weight and growth over the past year?
- Eat 5+ servings of fruits/vegetables a day; eat breakfast.
- Limit candy/soda/high-fat snacks.
- Get at least 2 cups low-fat milk/other dairy a day.
- Eat meals as a family.
- Be physically active 60 minutes a day.
  How often do you go outside to play?
- Limit screen time to 2 hours a day; no TV/computer in bedroom.
  How much time do you spend each day with TV or computers?

ORAL HEALTH

Regular visits with dentist, daily brushing and flossing, adequate fluoride

- Take child to dentist twice a year.
- Give fluoride supplement if dentist recommends.
- Brush teeth twice a day; floss once.
- Wear mouth guard during sports.

SAFETY

Knowing child's friends and their families, supervision with friends, safety belts/booster seats, helmets, playground safety, sports safety, swimming safety, sunscreen, smoke-free home/vehicles, guns, careful monitoring of computer use (games, Internet, e-mail)

- Know child's friends; teach home safety rules for fire/emergencies; teach rules for how to be safe with adults: (1) no adult should tell a child to keep secrets from parents, (2) no adult should express interest in private parts, (3) no adult should ask a child for help with his/her private parts.
  Do you know what to do if you get home and Mom or Dad are not there? What would you do if you felt unsafe at a friend's house? Has anyone touched you in a way that made you feel uncomfortable?

- Use belt-positioning booster seat in back seat until the lab/shoulder belt fits.
- Ensure child uses safety equipment (helmet, pads).
- Teach child to swim; supervise around water; use sunscreen.
- Keep home/vehicle smoke-free.
- Remove guns from home; if gun necessary, store unloaded and locked with ammunition locked separately.
- Monitor computer use; install safety filter.
  How much do you know about your child's Internet use? Do you have rules for the Internet?
  What would you do if you came to a site that scared you?

Key= Guidance for parent, *questions;* Guidance for child, *questions*

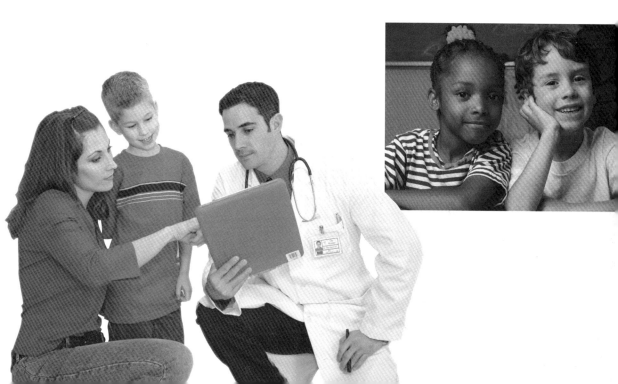

MIDDLE CHILDHOOD | 9 AND 10 YEAR VISITS

Observation of Parent-Child Interaction: Does parent allow child to talk with health care professional directly?

Surveillance of Development:
- Physical, cognitive, emotional, social, and moral competencies
- Behaviors that promote wellness and contribute to a healthy lifestyle
- Caring, supportive relationship with family, other adults, and peers
- Sense of self-confidence and hopefulness
- Increasingly responsible and independent decision making

Physical Exam. Complete, including: Measure blood pressure. Measure and plot height, weight. Calculate and plot BMI. Observe tattoos/piercings/signs of abuse, self-inflicted injuries. Note nevi or birthmarks. Examine back. Assess SMR.

Screening (See p 60.)

9 Year Visit
Universal: None
Selective: Vision; Hearing; Anemia; Tuberculosis

10 Year Visit
Universal: Vision; Hearing
Selective: Anemia; Tuberculosis; Dyslipidemia

Immunizations

CDC: www.cdc.gov/vaccines
AAP: www.aapredbook.org

38

Key= Guidance for parent, *questions;* Guidance for child, *questions*

Anticipatory Guidance

SCHOOL

School performance, homework, bullying

- Show interest in school performance and activities; if concerns, ask teacher about extra help.
  What are some things you are good at?
- Create quiet space for homework.
- Get help from teacher/trusted adult if bullied.

DEVELOPMENT AND MENTAL HEALTH

Emotional security and self-esteem, family communication and family time, temper problems and setting reasonable limits, friends, school performance, readiness for middle school, sexuality (pubertal onset, personal hygiene, initiation of growth spurt, menstruation and ejaculation, loss of "baby fat" and accretion of muscle, sexual safety)

- Promote independence, self-responsibility; assign chores; provide personal space at home.
- Be a positive role model; discuss respect, anger management.
- Know child's friends; supervise activities with peers.
  What do you and your friends like to do together? What do you do when friends pressure you to do things you don't want to do?
- Anticipate new adolescent behaviors, importance of peers.

- Answer questions about puberty/sexuality; counsel to avoid sexual activity; teach rules for how to be safe with adults: (1) no adult should tell a child to keep secrets from parents, (2) no adult should express interest in private parts, (3) no adult should ask a child for help with his/her private parts.
  How well do you and your partner agree on how to talk with your child about sexual development and sexuality? How would you respond if your child asked you about homosexuality?
  What questions do you have about the way your body is developing?

NUTRITION AND PHYSICAL ACTIVITY

Weight concerns, body image, importance of breakfast, limits on high-fat foods, water rather than soda or juice, eating as a family, physical activity

- Encourage nutritious food choices.
  What do you think of your child's weight and growth over the past year?
  What did you eat for breakfast today? Are you able to eat 5 or more fruits and vegetables every day? How do you feel about how you look? How often have you cut back on how much you eat or dieted to lose weight?
- Be physically active 60 minutes a day; limit non-academic screen time to 2 hours a day.
  How often do you go outside and play?

ORAL HEALTH

Regular visits with dentist, daily brushing and flossing, adequate fluoride

- Visit dentist twice a year.
- Give fluoride supplement if dentist recommends.
- Brush teeth twice a day; floss once.
- Wear mouth guard during sports.

SAFETY

Safety belts, helmets, bicycle safety, swimming, sunscreen, tobacco/alcohol/drugs, knowing child's friends and their families, supervision of child with friends, guns

- The back seat is the safest place to ride. Switch from booster seat to safety belt in rear seat, when the safety belt fits.
- Use safety equipment (helmets, pads).
- Teach child to swim, supervise around water; use sunscreen.
- Counsel about avoiding tobacco, alcohol, drugs.
  Is smoking, alcohol, or drug use a concern in your family? Is your child exposed to substance abuse?
- Know child's friends; make plan for personal safety.
  What would you do if you felt unsafe at a friend's house? Has anyone touched you in a way that made you feel uncomfortable?

- Remove guns from home; if gun necessary, store unloaded and locked with ammunition separate.
  Homicide and completed suicide are more common in homes with guns. Have you considered not owning a gun because it poses a danger to the family?
  What have your parents taught you about guns and gun safety?

Key= Guidance for parent, *questions;* Guidance for child, *questions*

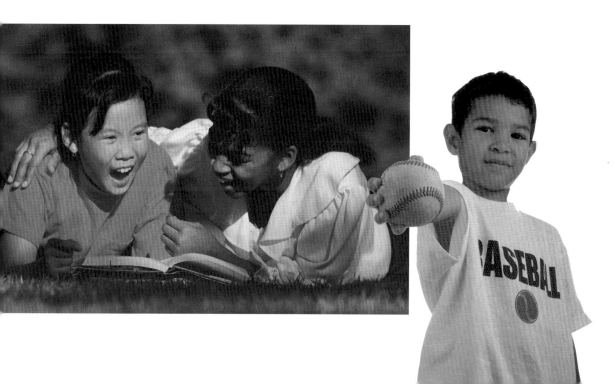

Observation of Parent-Youth Interaction: How comfortably do youth and parent interact? Who asks and answers most questions? Does youth express interest in managing his own health?

Surveillance of Development:
- Physical, cognitive, emotional, social, and moral competencies
- Behaviors that contribute to a healthy lifestyle
- Caring, supportive relationship with family, other adults, and peers
- Positive engagement with community
- Self-confidence, hopefulness, well-being, and resiliency when confronted with life stressors
- Increasingly responsible and independent decision making

Physical Exam. Complete, including: Measure blood pressure. Measure and plot height, weight. Calculate and plot BMI. Inspect for acne, acanthosis nigricans, atypical nevi, tattoos/piercings, signs of abuse or self-inflicted injury. Examine back. *Females:* Assess SMR; signs of STIs. Perform pelvic exam if warranted. *Males:* Observe for gynecomastia. Assess SMR, signs of STIs. Examine testicles for hydrocele, hernias, varicocele, masses.

Screening (See p 61.)

Universal: Vision (once in early adolescence)
Selective: Vision (when universal screening not performed); Hearing; Anemia; Tuberculosis; Dyslipidemia; STIs; Pregnancy; Cervical Dysplasia; Alcohol or Drug Use

Immunizations

CDC: www.cdc.gov/vaccines
AAP: www.aapredbook.org

Note: Beginning with the Early Adolescence Visits, many health care professionals conduct the first part of the medical interview with the parent in the examination room, and then spend time with the adolescent alone. This approach helps adolescents build a unique relationship with their health care professional, promotes confidence and full disclosure of health information, and enhances self-management. When explained within the context of healthy adolescent development, parents usually support this approach.

Key= Guidance for parent, *questions;* Guidance for youth, *questions*

Anticipatory Guidance

PHYSICAL GROWTH AND DEVELOPMENT

Physical and oral health, body image, healthy eating, physical activity

- Visit dentist twice a year; give fluoride supplement if dentist recommends.
- Brush teeth twice a day, floss once.
- Support healthy self-image by praising activities/achievements, not appearance.
- Encourage fruits/vegetables, whole grains, low-fat dairy; limit candy/chips/soda.
- Have 3+ servings low fat milk/other dairy a day; eat with your family.
- Be physically active 60 minutes a day; limit non-academic screen time to 2 hours a day.

SOCIAL AND ACADEMIC COMPETENCE

Connectedness with family, peers, and community; interpersonal relationships; school performance

- Clearly communicate rules/expectations/family responsibilities; spend time with your youth, get to know friends.
- Stay connected with family; follow family rules and curfews.

- Help youth follow their interests to new activities, increase awareness of community issues/needs.
- Explore interests and new activities, including those that help others.
- Praise positive efforts in school; help with organization/priority setting; encourage reading.
- Take responsibility for schoolwork; talk to parent/trusted adult about problems at school.

EMOTIONAL WELL-BEING

Coping, mood regulation and mental health, sexuality

- Involve youth in family decision making; encourage her to think through problems.
- Find ways to deal with stress.
- Tell me your concerns about your child's behavior, moods, mental health, or substance use.
  Do you have concerns about your child's emotional health?
- Everyone has difficult times and disappointments but usually they're temporary. Talk with parents/trusted adult/me if you are feeling sad, depressed, nervous, hopeless, or angry, especially if it makes it hard for you to keep on track with school, family, friends, and a generally positive attitude toward life.
  Have you been feeling bored, sad, or irritable most of the time? Do you ever feel so upset that you wished you were not alive or that you wanted to die?

- Youth go through puberty at different times; talk to your youth about the physical changes that occur during puberty, including menstruation for girls.
- Discuss your expectations/values about dating, relationships, and sex.
- Get accurate information about physical development, sexual feelings, and sexuality; talk to parents/trusted adult/me.
  For females: *Have you had your first period? If so, tell me more (how often, how heavy?)* For females and males: *Have you talked with your parents about dating and sex?*

RISK REDUCTION
Tobacco, alcohol, or other drugs; pregnancy; STIs

- Know youth's friends and activities; clearly discuss rules, expectations.
- Talk with youth about tobacco/alcohol/drugs; praise him for not using; be a role model.
- Consider locking liquor cabinet, putting prescription medicines in a place where youth cannot get them.
  Do you regularly supervise your child's social and recreational activities? What have you and your child discussed about the risk of using alcohol/tobacco/drugs?
- Don't smoke, drink, use drugs; avoid situations with drugs/alcohol; support friends who don't use; talk with me if concerned about your own, or a family member's, use.

Have you ever experimented with smoking/tobacco/alcohol/drugs/steroids? Do you ever sniff, "huff," or breathe anything to get high?

- Talk about relationships, sex, values; encourage sexual abstinence; provide opportunities for safe activities.
  How do you plan to help your child deal with pressures to have sex?
- The safest way to prevent pregnancy and STIs is to not have sex, including oral sex.
- Plan how to avoid risky situations; if sexually active, protect against STIs/pregnancy.
  Have you had sex? Was it wanted or unwanted? Have you ever been forced or pressured to do something sexual that you haven't wanted to do? Were your partners male or female, or have you had both male and female partners? Were your partners younger, older, or your age? Did you use a condom or other contraceptive?

VIOLENCE AND INJURY PREVENTION
Safety belt and helmet use, substance abuse and riding in a vehicle, guns, interpersonal violence (fights), bullying

- Wear safety belt; don't allow ATV riding.
- Wear safety belt, helmet, protective gear, life jacket.
- Help youth make plan for handling situation in which she feels unsafe riding in a car.
- Don't ride in car with driver who has used alcohol/drugs; call parents/trusted adult for help.
  Do you have someone you can call for a ride if you feel unsafe riding with someone?

Key= Guidance for parent, *questions;* Guidance for youth, *questions*

44

- Remove guns from home; if gun necessary, store unloaded and locked with ammunition locked separately.
  Homicide and completed suicide are more common in homes with guns. Have you considered not owning a gun because it poses a danger to the family?
  Do you ever carry a gun or knife?
- Healthy dating relationships are built on respect and concern; saying NO is okay.
  Have you ever been touched in a way that made you feel uncomfortable or was unwelcome? Have you ever been touched on your private parts against your wishes? Has anyone ever forced you to have sex?
- Teach nonviolent conflict-resolution techniques.
- Manage conflict nonviolently; talk to parent/trusted adult if bullied, stalked.

Observation of Parent-Youth Interaction: How comfortably do youth and parent interact? Who asks and answers most questions? Does youth express interest in managing his own health?

Surveillance of Development:
- Physical, cognitive, emotional, social, and moral competencies
- Behaviors that contribute to a healthy lifestyle
- Caring, supportive relationship with family, other adults, and peers
- Positive engagement with community
- Self-confidence, hopefulness, well-being, and resiliency when confronted with life stressors
- Increasingly responsible and independent decision making

Physical Exam. Complete, including: Measure blood pressure. Measure and plot height, weight. Calculate and plot BMI. Inspect for acne, acanthosis nigricans, atypical nevi, tattoos, piercings, signs of abuse or self-inflicted injury. Examine back. *Females:* Assess SMR, signs of STIs. Perform pelvic exam if warranted. *Males:* Observe for gynecomastia; SMR; signs of STIs. Examine testicles for hydrocele, hernias, varicocele, masses.

Screening (See p 61.)

Universal: Vision (once in middle adolescence)
Selective: Vision (when universal screening not performed); Hearing; Anemia; Tuberculosis; Dyslipidemia; STIs; Pregnancy; Cervical Dysplasia; Alcohol or Drug Use

Immunizations

CDC: www.cdc.gov/vaccines
AAP: www.aapredbook.org

Anticipatory Guidance

PHYSICAL GROWTH AND DEVELOPMENT

Physical and oral health, body image, healthy eating, physical activity

- Brush teeth twice a day; floss once.
- Visit dentist twice a year.
- Protect your hearing.
- Maintain healthy weight by balancing food choices/physical activity.
- Support healthy self-image by praising youth's activities/achievements, not appearance.
- Eat 3 meals a day, especially breakfast; focus on healthy food choices; have 3+ daily servings low-fat milk/other dairy; eat with your family.
- Encourage healthy eating.
- Be physically active 60 minutes a day; limit non-academic screen time to 2 hours a day.
- Encourage physical activity.

SOCIAL AND ACADEMIC COMPETENCE

Connectedness with family, peers, and community; interpersonal relationships; school performance

- Stay connected with family, help at home; get involved with community, friends; follow family rules (cars, curfews).
- Explore interests, new activities, including those that help others.
- Spend time with/praise youth; show affection; agree on limits, consequences; help youth follow interests to new activities, increase awareness of community issues/needs.
- Take responsibility for schoolwork; talk to parent/trusted adult about problems at school.
- Emphasize school, praise positive efforts, help with organization/priority setting, encourage reading.

EMOTIONAL WELL-BEING

Coping, mood regulation and mental health, sexuality

- Find ways to deal with stress; talk with parents/trusted adult.
- Involve youth in family decision making; encourage her to think through problems and practice independent decision making.
- Recognize that hard times come and go; talk with parents/trusted adult.
  Have you been feeling bored, sad, or irritable most of the time? Do you ever feel so upset that you wished you were not alive or that you wanted to die?
- Recognize signs of depression, anxiety or other mental health issues (irritability, changes in food/sleep habits, not adhering to rules, substance abuse).
  Do you have concerns about your youth's emotional health?

- Get accurate information about sexuality, physical development, sexual feelings; talk to parents/trusted adult/me.
  For females: Tell me about your periods (how often, how heavy, painful, most recent). For females and males: Have you talked with your parents about crushes you've had, about dating and relationships, and about sex? Do you have any questions related to physical development, sexuality, gender identity (your identity as a male or female), or sexual orientation? Have you had sex?
- Communicate frequently and share expectations clearly.

RISK REDUCTION
Tobacco, alcohol, or other drugs; pregnancy; STIs

- Don't smoke, drink, use drugs; avoid situations with drugs/alcohol; support friends who don't use; talk with me if you're concerned about family member's use.
  Have you ever experimented with smoking/tobacco/alcohol/drugs/steroids? Do you ever sniff, "huff," or breathe anything to get high?
- Talk with youth about tobacco/alcohol/drugs; know youth's friends and activities; clearly discuss rules/expectations; praise him for not using; be a role model; consider locking liquor cabinet, putting prescription medicines in a place where youth can't find them.
  Do you regularly supervise your youth's social and recreational activities? What have you and your youth discussed about the risk of using alcohol/tobacco/drugs?

- Abstaining from sexual intercourse, including oral sex, is the safest way to prevent pregnancy and STIs; plan how to avoid sex, risky situations.
- If sexually active, protect against STIs/pregnancy.
  Have you had sex? Was it wanted or unwanted? Have you ever felt pressured or forced to do something sexual that you didn't want to do? How many partners have you had in the past year? Were your partners male or female or have you had both male and female partners? Did you use a condom or other contraceptive?
- Encourage sexual abstinence; help youth make a plan for resisting pressure; support safe activities at school; talk about your values; have discussions with youth as she accepts responsibility for her decisions and relationships.
  Have you shared with your youth your hopes, expectations, and values about relationships and sex?

VIOLENCE AND INJURY PREVENTION
Safety belt and helmet use, driving (graduated license) and substance abuse, guns, interpersonal violence (dating violence), bullying

- Wear safety belt, helmet, protective gear, life jacket.
- Limit night driving, driving with teen passengers.
- Wear safety belt; be involved in youth's driving, set limits/expectations about number of passengers, night driving, distracted driving, high-risk situations.

Key= Guidance for youth, *questions;* Guidance for parent, *questions*

- Don't ride in car with driver who has used alcohol/ drugs; call parents/trusted adult for help; don't drink and drive.
  Do you have someone you can call for a ride if you feel unsafe riding with someone?
- Fighting, carrying weapons can be dangerous.
  Do you ever carry a gun? Is there a gun at home?
- Remove guns from home; if gun necessary, store un- loaded and locked with ammunition locked separately; keep key inaccessible to youth.
- Manage conflict nonviolently; avoid risky situations; healthy dating relationships are built on respect and doing things you both like to do; saying NO is okay.
- Teach nonviolent conflict-resolution techniques.

Observation of Parent-Young Adult Interaction:
How comfortably do young adult and parent, if present, interact? Is young adult appropriately encouraged to manage own health?

Surveillance of Development:
- Physical, cognitive, emotional, social, and moral competencies
- Behaviors that contribute to a healthy lifestyle
- Caring, supportive relationship with family, other adults, and peers
- Positive engagement with community
- Self-confidence, hopefulness, well-being, and resiliency when confronted with life stressors
- Increasingly responsible and independent decision making

Physical Exam. Complete, including: Measure blood pressure. Measure and plot height, weight. Calculate and plot BMI. Inspect for acne, acanthosis nigricans, atypical nevi, tattoos, piercings, signs of abuse or self-inflicted injury. *Females:* CBE routine after age 20. Assess signs of STIs. Perform pelvic exam if warranted. *Males:* Assess SMR; signs of STIs. Examine testicles for hydrocele, hernias, varicocele, masses.

Screening (See p 61.)

Universal: Vision (once in late adolescence); Dyslipidemia (once in late adolescence)
Selective screening: Vision (when universal screening not performed); Hearing; Anemia; Tuberculosis; Dyslipidemia (when universal screening not performed); STIs; Pregnancy; Cervical Dysplasia; Alcohol or Drug Use

Immunizations

CDC: www.cdc.gov/vaccines
AAP: www.aapredbook.org

50

Anticipatory Guidance

PHYSICAL GROWTH AND DEVELOPMENT

Physical and oral health, body image, healthy eating, physical activity

- Brush teeth twice a day, floss once; visit dentist twice a year.
- Protect your hearing.
- Eat 3 nutritious meals a day; fruits and vegetables; 3+ servings a day low-fat milk/other dairy.
- Be physically active 60 minutes a day, use protective gear; limit nonacademic screen time to 2 hours a day.

SOCIAL AND ACADEMIC COMPETENCE

Connectedness with family, peers, and community, interpersonal relationships, school performance

- Stay connected with family and friends; recognize some friendships change; get involved with community.
- Take responsibility for getting to school/work on time.
- Consider future education/work plans.
  What help do you need from me or your parents to help you reach your goal?

EMOTIONAL WELL-BEING

Coping, mood regulation and mental health, sexuality

- Find ways to deal with stress; practice problem solving and responsible/independent decision making.
- Recognize that most disappointments and setbacks are temporary; if you find that you are so sad, depressed, nervous, or angry that you can't get back on track with life, talk with parents/trusted adult/me.
  Have you been feeling bored, sad, or irritable most of the time? Do you ever feel so upset that you wished you were not alive or that you wanted to die?
- Sexuality is important to normal development as an adult.
  Do you have any questions related to physical development, sexuality, gender identity (your identity as a male or female), or sexual orientation? For females: Tell me about your periods (how often, how heavy, painful?).

RISK REDUCTION

Tobacco, alcohol, or other drugs, pregnancy, STIs

- Don't smoke, drink, use drugs/steroids/diet pills; avoid situations with drugs/alcohol; support friends who don't use.
  Tell me about any experiences you've had with alcohol, marijuana, or other drugs.

- Think through how to make sure you can carry out your decisions about sex. Considering role of alcohol and drug use and avoiding risky places and relationships can help.
- If sexually active, protect against STIs/pregnancy; make a plan so you can carry out your decisions about sex (avoid alcohol/risky situations).

  Have you had sex? Was it wanted or unwanted? Were your partners male or female or have you had both male and female partners? Did you use a condom or other contraceptive?

VIOLENCE AND INJURY PREVENTION

Safety belt and helmet use, substance abuse and riding in a vehicle, guns, interpersonal violence (fights), bullying

- Wear safety belt, helmet, protective gear, life jacket.
- Don't use alcohol/drugs and drive.
- Don't ride in car with driver who has used alcohol/drugs.
- Remove guns from home; if gun necessary, store unloaded and locked with ammunition separate; keep key away from any children.

  Do you ever carry a gun? Is there a gun at home?

- Manage conflict nonviolently; avoid risky situations; leave violent relationships; healthy relationships are built on respect, concern and mutual interests; saying NO is okay.

  Do you belong to a gang or know anyone in a gang? Have you ever been hit, slapped, or physically hurt while on a date? Have you ever been forced to have sexual intercourse?

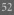

52

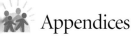

Appendices

Developmental Milestones at a Glance — Infancy
Developmental Milestones at a Glance — Early Childhood
Social and Emotional Development in Middle Childhood
Domains of Adolescent Development
Recommended Medical Screening — Infancy
Recommended Medical Screening — Early Childhood
Recommended Medical Screening — Middle Childhood
Recommended Medical Screening — Adolescence
Tooth Eruption Chart
Sexual Maturity Ratings
Useful Web Sites

Developmental Milestones at a Glance — Infancy

AGE	GROSS MOTOR	FINE MOTOR	COGNITIVE, LINGUISTIC, AND COMMUNICATION	SOCIAL-EMOTIONAL
2 Months	Head up 45° Lift head	Follow past midline Follow to midline	Laugh Vocalize	Smile spontaneously Smile responsively
4 Months	Roll over Sit—head steady	Follow to 180° Grasp rattle	Turn to rattling sound Laugh	Regard own hand
6 Months	Sit—no support Roll over	Look for dropped yarn Reach	Turn to voice Turn to rattling sound	Feed self Work for toy (out of reach)
9 Months	Pull to stand Stand holding on	Take 2 cubes Pass cube (transfer)	Dada/Mama, nonspecific Single syllables	Wave bye-bye Feed self

KEY

Black: 50% to 90% of children pass this item.

Green: More than 90% of children pass this item.

Source: See the Child Development theme in *Bright Futures: Guidelines for Health Supervision of Infants, Children, and Adolescents*, Third Edition.

Developmental Milestones at a Glance — Early Childhood

AGE	GROSS MOTOR	FINE MOTOR	COGNITIVE, LINGUISTIC, AND COMMUNICATION	SOCIAL-EMOTIONAL
1 Year	•Stand alone •Pull to stand	•Put block in cup •Bang 2 cubes held in hands	•Imitate vocalizations/sounds •Babbling* •1 word	•Protodeclarative pointing* •Wave bye-bye •Imitate activities •Play pat-a-cake
15 Months	•Walk backwards •Stoop and recover •Walk well	•Scribble •Put block in cup	•1 word* •3 words	•Drink from cup •Wave bye-bye
18 Months	•Walk up steps •Run •Walk backwards	•Dump raisin, demonstrated •Tower of 2 cubes •Scribble	•Point to at least 1 body part •6 words •3 words	•Remove garment •Help in house
2 Years	•Throw ball overhand •Jump up •Kick ball forward •Walk up steps	•Tower of 6 cubes •Tower of 4 cubes	•Name 1 picture •Combine words •Point to 2 pictures	•Put on clothing •Remove garment
2½ Years	•Throw ball overhand •Jump up	•Imitate vertical line •Tower of 8 cubes •Tower of 6 cubes	•Know 2 actions •Speech half understandable •Point to 6 body parts •Name 1 picture	•Wash and dry hands •Put on clothing
3 Years	•Balance on each foot 1 second •Broad jump •Throw ball overhand	•Thumb wiggle •Imitate vertical line •Tower of 8 cubes •Tower of 6 cubes	•Speech all understandable •Name 1 color •Know 2 adjectives •Name 4 pictures	•Name friend •Brush teeth with help
4 Years	•Hop •Balance on each foot 2 seconds	•Draw a person with 3 parts •Tower of 8 cubes	•Define 5 words •Name 4 colors •Speech all understandable	•Copy a cross (+) •Copy a circle

KEY

Black: 50% to 90% of children pass this item.

Green: More than 90% of children pass this item.

*Absence of this milestone should trigger screening for autism.

Source: See the Child Development theme in *Bright Futures: Guidelines for Health Supervision of Infants, Children, and Adolescents*, Third Edition.

Social and Emotional Development in Middle Childhood

TOPICS	KEY AREAS (Key areas in italics are especially important for children with special health care needs.)
Self	Self-esteem: • Experiences of success • Reasonable risk-taking behavior • Resilience and ability to handle failure • Supportive family and peer relationships Self-image: • Body image, *celebrating different body images* • Prepubertal changes; initiating discussion about sexuality and reproduction; *prepubertal changes related to physical care issues*
Family	What matters at home: • Expectation and limit setting • Family times together • Communication • Family responsibilities • Family transitions • Sibling relationships • *Caregiver relationships*
Friends	Friendships: • Making friends, *friendships with peers with and without special health care needs* • Family support of friendships, *family support to have typical friendship activities, as appropriate*
School	School: • Expectation for school performance, *school performance/defined in the Individualized Education Program* • Homework • Child-teacher conflicts, *building relationships with teachers* • *Parent-teacher communication* • Ability of schools to address the needs of children from diverse backgrounds • Awareness of aggression, bullying, and victimization • Absenteeism
Community	Community strengths: • Community organizations • Religious groups • Cultural groups High-risk behaviors and environments: • Substance use • Unsafe friendships • Unsafe community environments • *Particular awareness of risk-taking behaviors and unsafe environments, because children may be easily victimized*

Source: See the Child Development theme in *Bright Futures: Guidelines for Health Supervision of Infants, Children, and Adolescents*, Third Edition.

Domains of Adolescent Development

	EARLY ADOLESCENCE (11 TO 14 YEARS)	MIDDLE ADOLESCENCE (15 TO 17 YEARS)	LATE ADOLESCENCE (18 TO 21 YEARS)
Physiological	Onset of puberty, growth spurt, menarche (females)	Ovulation (females), growth spurt (males)	Growth completed
Psychological	Concrete thought, preoccupation with rapid body changes, sexual identity, questioning independence, parental controls remain strong	Competence in abstract and future thought, idealism, sense of invincibility or narcissism, sexual identity, beginning of cognitive capacity to provide legal consent	Future orientation, emotional independence, unmasking of psychiatric disorders, capacity for empathy, intimacy, and reciprocity in interpersonal relationships, self-identity; recognized as legally capable of providing consent, attainment of legal age for some issues (eg, voting) but not all issues (eg, drinking alcohol)
Social	Search for same-sex peer affiliation, good parental relationships, other adults as role models; transition to middle school, involvement in extracurricular activities; sensitivity to differences between home culture and culture of others	Beginning emotional emancipation, increased power of peer group, conflicts over parental control, interest in sexual relationships, initiation of driving, risk-taking behavior, transition to high school, reduced involvement in extracurricular activities; possible cultural conflict as adolescent navigates between family's values and values of broader culture and peer culture	Individual over peer relationships; transition in parent-child relationship, transition out of home; may begin preparation for further education, career, marriage, and parenting
Potential Problems	Delayed puberty, acne, orthopedic problems, school problems, psychosomatic concerns, depression, unintended pregnancy; initiation of tobacco, alcohol, or other drug use	Experimentation with health risk behaviors (eg, sex, drinking, drug use, smoking), auto crashes, menstrual disorders, unintended pregnancy, acne, short stature (males), conflicts with parents, overweight, physical inactivity, poor eating behaviors, eating disorders (eg, purging, binge eating, and anorexia nervosa)	Eating disorders, depression, suicide, auto crashes, unintended pregnancy, acne, smoking, alcohol or drug dependence

Source: See the Child Development theme in *Bright Futures: Guidelines for Health Supervision of Infants, Children, and Adolescents,* Third Edition.

Recommended Medical Screening — Infancy

UNIVERSAL	ACTION	NB	1W	1M	2M	4M	6M	9M
Metabolic and hemoglobinopathy	Done according to state law	•	•	•	•			
Development	Structured developmental screen							•
Oral health	Administer OH risk assessment						•	•
Hearing	All NB before discharge; if not by discharge, in 1st month; verify documentation of screening results and appropriate rescreening by 2M		•	•	•	•		

SELECTIVE	RISK ASSESSMENT (RA)	ACTION IF RA +	NB	1W	1M	2M	4M	6M	9M
Blood pressure	Children with specific risk conditions or change in risk	Blood pressure	•	•	•	•	•	•	•
Vision	Prematurity with risk conditions, abnormal fundoscopic exam, parental concern (all visits); abnormal eye alignment (4M and 6M); abnormal cover/uncover test (9M)	Ophthalmology referral	•	•	•	•	•	•	•
Hearing	+ on risk screening questions	Referral for diagnostic audiologic assessment						•	•
Anemia	Preterm/LBW; not on iron-fortified formula	Hemoglobin or hematocrit					•		
Lead	+ on risk screening questions	Lead screen						•	•
Tuberculosis	+ on risk screening questions	Tuberculin skin test			•			•	

OH = oral health; **NB** = newborn; **LBW** = low birth weight

Recommended Medical Screening — Early Childhood

UNIVERSAL	ACTION	12M	15M	18M	2Y	2½Y	3Y	4Y
Development	Structured developmental screen			•		•		
Autism	Autism Specific Screen			•	•			
Vision	Objective measure with age-appropriate visual acuity measurement (using HOTV; tumbling E tests; Snellen letters; Snellen numbers; or Picture tests, such as Allen figures or LEA symbols)						•	•
Hearing	Audiometry							•
Anemia	Hematocrit or hemoglobin	•						
Lead*	Lead screen	•			•			

SELECTIVE	RISK ASSESSMENT (RA)	ACTION IF RA +	12M	15M	18M	2Y	2½Y	3Y	4Y
Oral health	No dental home	Referral to dental home; if not available, oral health risk assessment (12M, 18M, 2Y, 2½Y). Referral to dental home (3Y).	•		•	•	•	•	
	Primary water source is deficient in fluoride	Oral fluoride supplementation	•		•	•	•	•	•
Blood pressure†	Specific risk conditions or change in risk	Blood pressure	•	•	•	•	•		
Vision	Parental concern or abnormal fundoscopic exam or cover/uncover test	Ophthalmology referral	•	•	•	•	•		
Hearing	+ on risk screening questions	Referral for diagnostic audiologic assessment	•	•	•	•	•	•	
Anemia	+ on risk screening questions	Hematocrit or hemoglobin			•	•	•	•	•
Lead‡	+ on risk screening questions	Lead screen	•			•			
Lead	No previous screen or change in risk	Lead screen				•			
	No previous screen and + on risk screening questions or change in risk	Lead screen						•	•
Tuberculosis	+ on risk screening questions	Tuberculin skin test	•		•	•	•	•	•
Dyslipidemia	+ on risk screening questions; not previously screened with normal results (4Y)	Fasting lipid profile				•			•

*Universal lead screen = high prevalence area or on Medicaid; †Beginning at age 3, blood pressure becomes part of the physical examination; ‡Selective lead screen = low prevalence area and not on Medicaid.

Recommended Medical Screening — Middle Childhood

UNIVERSAL	ACTION		5Y	6Y	7Y	8Y	9Y	10Y
Vision	Objective measure with age-appropriate visual acuity measurement (using HOTV; tumbling E tests; Snellen letters; Snellen numbers; or Picture tests, such as Allen figures or LEA symbols)		•	•				
	Snellen test					•		•
Hearing	Audiometry		•	•		•		•
SELECTIVE	RISK ASSESSMENT (RA)	ACTION IF RA +	5Y	6Y	7Y	8Y	9Y	10Y
Oral health	No dental home	Referral to dental home		•				
	Primary water source deficient in fluoride	Oral fluoride supplementation		•				
Vision	+ on risk screening questions	Snellen test			•		•	
Hearing	+ on risk screening questions	Audiometry			•		•	
Anemia	+ on risk screening questions	Hemoglobin or hematocrit	•	•	•	•	•	•
Lead	No previous screen and + on risk screening questions or change in risk	Lead screen	•	•				
Tuberculosis	+ on risk screening questions	Tuberculin skin test	•	•	•	•	•	•
Dyslipidemia	+ on risk screening questions and not previously screened with normal results	Fasting lipid profile		•		•		•

Recommended Medical Screening — Adolescence

UNIVERSAL	ACTION		EARLY (11-14Y)	MIDDLE (15-17Y)	LATE (18-21Y)
Vision (once during each age stage)	Snellen test		•	•	•
Dyslipidemia (once during Late Adolescence)	A fasting lipoprotein profile (total cholesterol, LDL cholesterol high density lipoprotein [hDL], cholesterol and triglyceride). If the testing opportunity is non-fasting, only total cholesterol and HDL cholesterol will be usable.				•
SELECTIVE	**RISK ASSESSMENT (RA)**	**ACTION IF RA +**	EARLY (11-14Y)	MIDDLE (15-17Y)	LATE (18-21Y)
Vision (when universal screening not performed)	+ on risk screening questions	Snellen test	•	•	•
Hearing	+ on risk screening questions	Audiometry	•	•	•
Anemia	+ on risk screening questions	Hemoglobin or hematocrit	•	•	•
Tuberculosis	+ on risk screening questions	Tuberculin skin test	•	•	•
Dyslipidemia (when universal screening not performed)	+ on risk screening questions and not previously screened with normal results	Lipid screen	•	•	•
STIs	Sexually active	Chlamydia and gonorrhea screen; use tests appropriate to the patient population and clinical setting	•	•	•
	Sexually active and + on risk screening questions	Syphilis blood test HIV*	•	•	•
Pregnancy	Sexually active without contraception, late menses, amenorrhea, or heavy or irregular bleeding	Urine hCG	•	•	•
Cervical dysplasia	Sexually active, within 3 years of onset of sexual activity or no later than age 21	Pap smear, conventional slide or liquid-based	•	•	•
Alcohol or drug use	+ on risk screening questions	Administer alcohol- and drug-screening tool	•	•	•

*The CDC has recently recommended universal voluntary HIV screening for all sexually active people, beginning at age 13. At the time of publication, the AAP and other groups had not yet commented on the CDC recommendation, nor recommended screening criteria or techniques. The health care professional's attention is drawn to the voluntary nature of screening and that the CDC allows an opt out in communities where the HIV rate is <0.1%. The management of positives and false positives must be considered before testing.

Tooth Eruption Chart

Primary Dentition

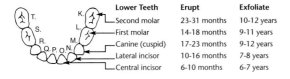

Upper Teeth	Erupt	Exfoliate
Central incisor	8-12 months	6-7 years
Lateral incisor	9-13 months	7-8 years
Canine (cuspid)	16-22 months	10-12 years
First molar	13-19 months	9-11 years
Second molar	25-33 months	10-12 years

Lower Teeth	Erupt	Exfoliate
Second molar	23-31 months	10-12 years
First molar	14-18 months	9-11 years
Canine (cuspid)	17-23 months	9-12 years
Lateral incisor	10-16 months	7-8 years
Central incisor	6-10 months	6-7 years

Permanent Dentition

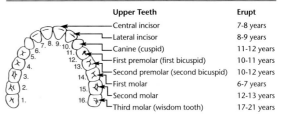

Upper Teeth	Erupt
Central incisor	7-8 years
Lateral incisor	8-9 years
Canine (cuspid)	11-12 years
First premolar (first bicuspid)	10-11 years
Second premolar (second bicuspid)	10-12 years
First molar	6-7 years
Second molar	12-13 years
Third molar (wisdom tooth)	17-21 years

Lower Teeth	Erupt
Third molar (wisdom tooth)	17-21 years
Second molar	12-13 years
First molar	6-7 years
Second premolar (second bicuspid)	10-12 years
First premolar (first bicuspid)	10-11 years
Canine (cuspid)	11-12 years
Lateral incisor	8-9 years
Central incisor	7-8 years

Source: Reproduced with permission from the Arizona Department of Health Services, Office of Oral Health, courtesy of Don Altman, DDS, MPH.
The assistance of the American Dental Hygienists' Association is gratefully acknowledged.

Sexual Maturity Ratings

Sexual maturity ratings (SMRs) are widely used to assess adolescents' physical development during puberty in 5 stages (from preadolescent to adult). Also known as Tanner stages, SMRs are a way of assessing the degree of maturation of secondary sexual characteristics.

The developmental stages of the adolescent's sexual characteristics should be rated separately (ie, one stage for pubic hair and one for breasts in females, one stage for pubic hair and one for genitals in males), because these characteristics may differ in their degree of maturity.

Sexual Maturity Ratings: Males

SMR	PUBIC HAIR
Stage 1	None
Stage 2	Scanty, long, slightly pigmented, primarily at base of penis
Stage 3	Darker, courser, starts to curl, small amount
Stage 4	Course, curly; resembles adult type but covers smaller area
Stage 5	Adult quantity and distribution, spread to medial surface of thighs

SMR	GENITALS	
	PENIS	TESTES
Stage 1	Preadolescent	Preadolescent
Stage 2	Slight enlargement	Slight enlargement of testes and scrotum; scrotal skin reddened, texture altered
Stage 3	Longer	Further enlargement of testes and scrotum
Stage 4	Larger in breadth, glans penis develops	Further enlargement of testes and scrotum
Stage 5	Adult	Adult

Sexual Maturity Ratings: Females

SMR	PUBIC HAIR
Stage 1	None
Stage 2	Sparse, slightly pigmented, straight, at medial border of labia
Stage 3	Darker, beginning to curl, increased amount
Stage 4	Course, curly, abundant, but amount less than in adult
Stage 5	Adult feminine triangle, spread to medial surface of thighs

SMR	BREASTS
Stage 1	Preadolescent
Stage 2	Breast and papilla elevated as small mound; areolar diameter increased
Stage 3	Breast and areola enlarged, no contour separation
Stage 4	Areola and papilla form secondary mound
Stage 5	Mature; nipple projects, areola part of general breast contour

Source: Tables have been adapted with permission from Daniels[1(p79)] (as drawn from Tanner[2]); see also Spear.[3(p4)]

References

1. Daniels WA. *Adolescents in Health and Disease.* St Louis, MO: Mosby, Inc; 1977

2. Tanner JM. *Growth at Adolescence.* 2nd ed. Oxford, England: Blackwell Scientific Publications; 1962

3. Spear B. *Adolescent growth and development.* In: Rickert VI, ed. *Adolescent Nutrition: Assessment and Management.* New York, NY: Chapman and Hall (Aspen Publishers, Inc); 1996:3-24

Useful Web Sites

American Academy of Pediatrics
www.aap.org

American Academy of Pediatrics Bright Futures
http://brightfutures.aap.org

American Academy of Pediatrics Clinical Guide:
Connected Kids
www.aap.org/ConnectedKids/ClinicalGuide.pdf

American Academy of Pediatrics *Red Book Online*
www.aapredbook.org

American Association of Poison Control Centers
(Poison Control: 800-222-1222 and 911)
www.aapcc.org

American College of Obstetricians and Gynecologists
www.acog.org

Automotive Safety Program
www.preventinjury.org

Centers for Disease Control and Prevention
Morbidity and Mortality Weekly Report
www.cdc.gov/mmwr/pdf/ss/ss5505.pdf

Centers for Disease Prevention and Control
National Immunization Program
www.cdc.gov/vaccines

Centers for Disease Control and Prevention
National Immunization Information Hotline
(800-CDC-INFO)
www.vaccines.ashastd.org

Centers for Disease Prevention and Control
Physical Activity for Everyone
www.cdc.gov/nccdphp/dnpa/physical/recommendations/
young.htm

Child Safety Seat Information
(866-SEATCHECK [866-732-8243])
www.seatcheck.org

Institute of Medicine of the National Academies
www.iom.edu/file.asp?id=21372

Maternal and Child Health Bureau
Accurately Weighing & Measuring: Technique
http://depts.washington.edu/growth/module5/text/
contents.htm

MyPyramid, US Department of Agriculture
www.mypyramid.gov/kids/index.html

National Association for Sport & Physical Education
www.aahperd.org/naspe/template.cfm?template=
toddlers.html

National Cancer Institute Smoking Cessation Information
(1-800-QUITNOW)
http://1800quitnow.cancer.gov

National Center for Education Statistics
www.nces.ed.gov

National Center for Health Statistics
www.cdc.gov/nchs

National Center for Health Statistics Growth Charts
www.cdc.gov/growthcharts

National Center for Homeless Education
www.serve.org/nche

National Guideline Clearinghouse
www.guideline.gov

National Institute of Mental Health
www.nimh.nih.gov

National Maternal and Child Oral Health Resource Center
www.mchoralhealth.org

National Society of Genetic Counselors
www.nsgc.org/consumer/familytree

National Youth Violence Prevention Resource Center
www.safeyouth.org

Olweus Bullying Prevention Program
www.clemson.edu/olweus/index.html

Reach Out and Read
www.reachoutandread.org

Safe Kids Worldwide
www.safekids.org/members/unitedStates.html

Statistical Abstract of the United States
www.census.gov/prod/www/statistical-abstract.html

The Cochrane Collaboration
www.cochrane.org

The National Early Childhood Technical Assistance Center
www.nectac.org/topics/earlyid/partcelig.asp

The President's Council on Physical Fitness and Sports
http://fitness.gov

US Department of Health & Human Services
Guide to Reliable Health Information
www.healthfinder.gov

US Department of Labor
http://jobcorps.doleta.gov

Web-based Injury Statistics Query and Reporting System
www.cdc.gov/ncipc/wisqars

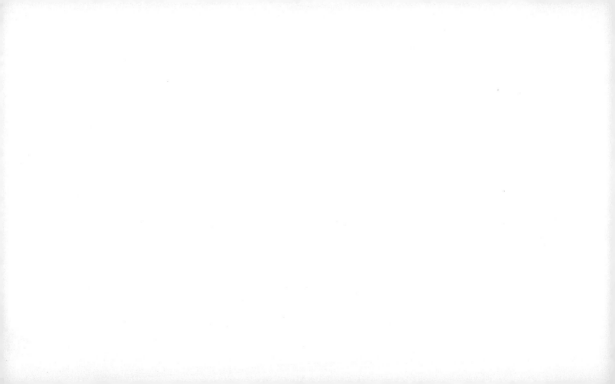